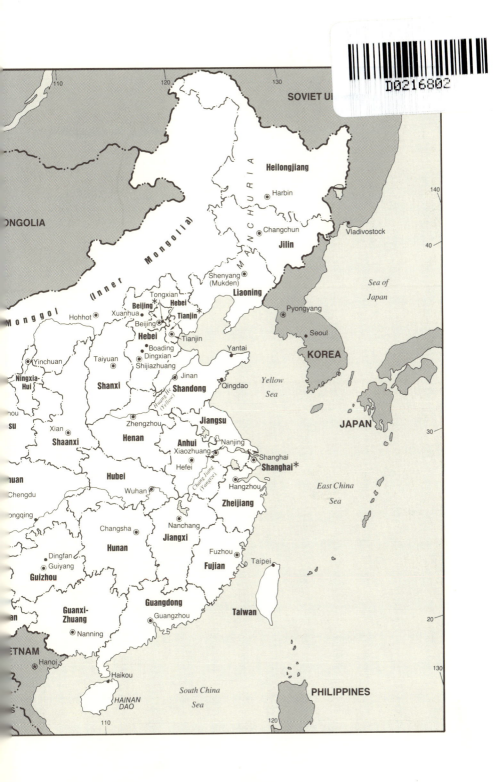

SOVIET U[N]

MONGOLIA

(Inner Mongolia)

Monggol

Heilongjiang

Harbin

Changchun

Jilin

MANCHURIA

Vladivostock

140

40

Sea of
Japan

Shenyang (Mukden)

Liaoning

Pyongyang

Seoul

KOREA

Hohhot

Xuanhua

Beijing
Beijing

Tongxian

Hebei

Tianjin
Tianjin

Hebei

Boading

Dingxian

Shijiazhuang

Yantai

JAPAN

30

Yinchuan

Ningxia-Hui

Taiyuan

Shanxi

Jinan

Shandong

Qingdao

*Yellow
Sea*

Huang He
(Yellow)

Xian

Shaanxi

Zhengzhou

Henan

Jiangsu

Nanjing

Anhui
Xiaozhuang

Hefei

Shanghai

Shanghai

*East China
Sea*

Chengdu

ongqing

Hubei

Wuhan

Chang Jiang
(Yangtze)

Hangzhou

Zheijiang

Changsha

Nanchang

Jiangxi

Hunan

Dingfan

Guiyang

Guizhou

Fuzhou

Fujian

Taipei

Taiwan

Guangdong

Guangzhou

20

130

Guanxi-Zhuang

Nanning

PHILIPPINES

ETNAM

Hanoi

Haikou

*HAINAN
DAO*

*South China
Sea*

110

120

30

Medicine in Rural China

Medicine in Rural China

A Personal Account

C. C. Chen, M.D.

in collaboration with
Frederica M. Bunge

University of California Press

Berkeley · Los Angeles · London

University of California Press
Berkeley and Los Angeles, California

University of California Press, Ltd.
London, England

Copyright © 1989 by
The Regents of the University of California

Library of Congress Cataloging in Publication Data

Chen, C. C., 1903–
    Medicine in rural China : a personal account / C.C. Chen, in collaboration with
Frederica M. Bunge.
        p.   cm.
    Bibliography: p.
    Includes index.
    ISBN 0-520-06298-1 (alk. paper)

    1. Medical care—China.   2. Public health—China.   I. Bunge,
Frederica M.   II. Title.
    [DNLM: 1. Medicine, Chinese Traditional—history—China—personal
narratives.   2. Public Health—history—China—personal narratives.
3. Rural Health—history—China—personal narratives. WA 11 JC6 C5m]
RA527.C49   1989
610'.951—dc19
DNLM/DLC
for Library of Congress   88-17223
                                                                                CIP

Printed in the United States of America

1 2 3 4 5 6 7 8 9

To Betty and Jim,
in memory of their father,
John B. Grant, M.D.

Contents

Foreword

The sixty years spanned by these memoirs in community medicine have witnessed more progress in the health of people than the preceding 2,000 years. Worldwide infant mortality rates have been more than halved and life expectancy nearly doubled.

When Dr. C. C. Chen started his medical studies in the 1920s, few states saw the health of their citizens as a responsibility of government. By 1985, it was possible for the World Health Organization and the United Nations Children's Fund to talk seriously of universal immunization for children by 1990, of the potential for a virtual child survival revolution in many developing countries before the close of the 1990s, and of the possibility of achieving health for all by the year 2000 through primary health care.

When we explore how this transformation was possible, we see that the reasons are complex; we also see a handful of intellectual giants to whom the world community owes a deep debt of gratitude for their articulation and demonstration of the basic concepts now known as primary health care.

C. C. Chen is one of these.

His memoirs are unique, not only in the length of time they span but also in the breadth of firsthand experience with primary health care that they encompass.

C. C. Chen was one of the pioneers in systematically addressing the immediate social problem of overtaking the lag between modern medical knowledge and its use in a low-income community. It was in the county of Dingxian, with a largely rural population of more than 100,000, that C. C. Chen introduced the use of the scientific method to bear on addressing this lag in a low-income rural setting. In a period of a few years, he and his colleagues, working closely with Dr. James Yen and the Mass Education Movement that had come earlier to Dingxian, demonstrated dramatically successful techniques, including methods for involving villagers in improving their own health condition. The major principles they established then, described in these memoirs, have proved to be remarkably durable over the past half century and a remarkable testament to Dr. Chen and his colleagues.

One can only wish that the world community had been quicker to accept these scientific principles of sound organization so convincingly demonstrated then, including the facts that:

- The use of medical knowledge and the efficiency of health protection depend chiefly upon sound organization.
- A vertical medical system cannot stand by itself unless it is integrated with other social activities in a joint horizontal attack on the problems of social reconstruction.
- Demonstration units must take into consideration the economic practicability of extending them to the nation as a whole. This implies that the principle of self-help, or participation by the consumer, be adopted, as no low-income country can afford to make full use of available medical knowledge through tax funds alone.

As becomes apparent soon to a reader of these memoirs, C. C. Chen was first a student and later a colleague of the late Dr. John B. Grant, my father, then Professor of Public Health at the Rockefeller-endowed Peking Union Medical College. It was my privilege to accompany my father on a visit to Dingxian in 1934. John Grant was one of the early pioneers in international health and in bringing medical knowledge to the benefit of populations as a whole. C. C. Chen undertook his initial work in public health at Dingxian at the urging of Dr. Grant, and Dingxian was used as an influential training ground for many of the medical students at this preeminent medical institution of the 1930s. Their visitors included men who were to leave their mark on world health in other ways. These included Dr. Andrija Stampar, the Yugoslav pioneer in rural health who later was to become the first chairman of the World Health Organization (WHO), and Dr. Ludwig Rajchman, the Pole who was then Director of the Health Bureau of the League of Nations, the predecessor to WHO, and who was, after World War II, to become the founder and chairman for the first five years of the organization I now serve as Executive Director, the United Nations Children's Fund (UNICEF). These men all belonged to a generation who believed, to paraphrase Professor Toynbee, that theirs was the first generation for which it was possible to conceive of bringing the benefits of civilization to all humankind.

The 1937 Japanese invasion of China brought the Dingxian experiment to an untimely end. Fortunately, knowledge of this experiment was already beginning to be applied in many parts of China and was later to contribute to the extraordinary progress China has made since 1950 in improving the health of its people.

With a per capita income of probably still less than that of the United States two centuries ago, China by the 1980s has achieved a level of health in its population, when measured in terms of infant mortality rate and life expectancy, which approximates that of the United States at mid-twentieth century. If all developing countries had achieved the health conditions that China has achieved, some 8 million fewer children under the age of five years would have died (and there would have been 40 million fewer births) each year in the late 1980s. In achieving this, China has demonstrated the validity of principles first scientifically tested at Dingxian: that primary health care must involve popular participation to be successful, and a vertical medical system cannot be truly effective, or even stand by itself, unless it is integrated with other activities in a joint attack on the problems of development and social reconstruction. Primary health care must encompass education for health, adequate food and nutrition, clean water, and shelter and clothing for protection from the environment. We have seen in China that health is not simply a "sector" but also an explicit goal to be achieved through all sectors with mass participation.

It is also notable that what John Grant and C. C. Chen learned together in China had a major impact in Europe. When John Grant went to Europe as international health advisor for the Rockefeller Foundation in the immediate postwar years, the basic principles that were hammered out in China through use of scientific methods proved to be applicable also to the more developed countries of Europe.

Many of the European countries were then in the process of revising their health systems so that the first mass applications of these principles were effective in Europe rather than China. When my father left Europe after several years, government after government honored him with decorations—from Finland in the north to France in the south—for his advice drawn from his experience with his colleagues in China and India.

Dr. C. C. Chen offers one more invaluable service to the world by sharing with us these memoirs of a lifetime dedicated to promoting the health of peoples. In reading them, one is conscious of the fact that full application of the principles developed fifty years ago at Dingxian could still bring substantial improvements in health and well-being in China as well as much larger improvements in most other developing countries. There is much to be gained even today from application of the lessons of his experience in seeking to overtake the far-too-long lag between the development of modern knowledge and its use in the setting of a low-income community.

James P. Grant

Preface

T his book, perhaps more than most, requires a preface in order to avoid any serious misconceptions on the part of the reader. Although the book is being published by a university press, it is not a major work of research in the usual sense. It is told in the first person but is actually the product of collaboration between two individuals working at a distance from each other. Because of the specific nature of the collaboration, the reader should be warned against assuming that the attitudes and perspectives or views and interpretations expressed or implied throughout the book are unvaryingly those of its author, C. C. Chen, M.D. Emphatically, this is not the case. Material from Western sources, with its own theoretical and ideological perspectives, has been added to the draft. It is thus useful, probably even essential, for the reader to begin exploration of this volume with a clear knowledge of how the manuscript evolved and the ground it is intended to cover.

The author, a scientifically trained physician, was born in China in 1903 and lives there today with most of his family. As teacher, scholar, and administrator, he has moved repeatedly in and out of academic settings during his long career and presently holds the ranks of professor of community medicine at a key medical college.

During his long career, spanning some sixty years, Dr. Chen has enjoyed a number of opportunities to study and travel outside his own country. For example, he earned the degree of Master of Public Health at Harvard University in the academic year 1930/31 and has returned to the United States several times since. In 1985, after obtaining permission from Chinese authorities to come to the United States to write his memoirs, he spent several months on the campus of the University of California, Berkeley, where he devoted himself to that task. He wrote in English, a language he speaks fluently.

Dr. Chen had already completed the original draft of his text when Joyce C. Lashof, M.D., Dean of the School of Public Health, brought us together. I had just completed a master's program at the school and, before coming to Berkeley, had been chairperson of the Asia Research Team at the American University in Washington, D.C. for eight years. In that capacity I had coauthored more than a dozen multidisciplinary studies on Asian countries, including a 600-page 1980 China study. Dr. Lashof believed, therefore, that I was particularly qualified to lend editorial support to Dr. Chen's projected work.

In writing the original draft, Dr. Chen, who is first and foremost a medical scientist, had omitted almost all reference to the major historic events that provided the backdrop to the events in his life. Those who read that first version appreciated his devotion to his central topic. At the same time, they agreed that a certain amount of contextual material was necessary as the author wished to be heard internationally as well as at home. It could not be assumed that in a worldwide audience of health workers, all readers would necessarily be knowledgeable about events and conditions in China before and after liberation in 1949. So the matter was discussed with Dr. Chen, and it was agreed that some broadly descriptive material on economic and political conditions, institutions, and patterns of behavior would be included in order to provide the needed historical perspective.

Our collaboration began in December 1985 and continued over the succeeding two years. Having read the original manuscript with great care, I met with Dr. Chen in his campus office over a period of several weeks, as we discussed his personal philosophy and his goals and objectives in writing the book. The next month Dr. Chen returned to China, following lens-implant surgery. After reading the draft once again and reflecting on our taped conversations, I submitted a lengthy tentative outline for a new draft, and after he had approved that draft with some minor changes, revised and recast the existing text in accordance with it and added other major segments.

In August 1986 Dr. Chen arranged for me to spend two weeks with him at West China Union University of Medical Sciences in Chengdu, where we engaged in a fruitful exchange, going over the second draft line by line, agreeing on certain further changes as well as the addition of new material regarding important developments that had taken place in public health in early- to mid-1986. After returning to the United States, I revised the introduction and the chapters to varying degrees once again and prepared the seventh and final analytical chapter of the memoirs. By further correspondence, we worked out the details of this third and final draft, which was finalized and submitted to the publisher in January 1987. To make the work as timely as possible, we updated some points even after the book was accepted for publication late in 1987.

As to the material added to the text in the course of our collaboration, most of it is found in the historical setting components of each of the chronological chapters and in the Postliberation portion of the book as a whole. As I am not a specialist on East Asia or China, I collected the material largely from readily available English-language sources in Western libraries, particularly that of the graduate library at the University of California, Berkeley.

The implications of that latter fact are critical to the readers' understanding and assessment of these memoirs. Western and Chinese scholars will often have widely differing interpretations of the same data, the same circumstances, and the same events; as Dr. Chen is Chinese, he presumably shares the Chinese perspective. At certain points in the text, therefore, a careful reader might want to distinguish between assertions made by the author himself and those interposed by someone else. This should not necessarily be very difficult; the assertions of the author are those of a medically informed person.

Every effort has been made to bring to Dr. Chen's attention certain passages for which he was not directly responsible; however, it cannot be said with absolute certainty that this was always the case. We had to interact through correspondence, and a process of continuing revision was being carried out. Moreover, as time passed, Dr. Chen experienced increasing visual impairment, putting him at a severe disadvantage as he was unable to read for extended periods without experiencing severe eyestrain.

Dr. Chen might have chosen to produce either a work of original research or an academic treatise on which he could engage in critical debate with other scholars in the field. Such an approach would, however, have been entirely inconsistent with the beliefs and principles to which he has adhered so strongly all his life. In fact, Dr. Chen's international renown as a physician and a pioneer in the Chinese health experience is attributable to his lifelong commitment to action and intervention, manifest especially in his experimentation with the development of a rural health system at Dingxian in North China during the 1930s. North China constituted the northern part of so-called China proper—eighteen historic provinces within the Great Wall. Given this commitment, along with his emphasis on educational experience "in the field," it is in no way surprising that he has written a very different kind of book. Instead of speaking to an academic audience, he is addressing health activists, educators, trainers, and primary health care workers, especially those in the Third World, sharing with them the story of a humanistic attempt to find practical ways of introducing scientific medicine for people living under difficult conditions.

Sensitively aware of the limitations of his own knowledge and of the diversity of his country and its propensity for rapid change, the author has tried to confine this study to issues and problems with which he has had firsthand experience, eschewing any suggesting that what he describes in his own province or county necessarily pertains to China as a whole. As a result, we are treated to a strictly personal account of rural health development, focusing on districts and counties where Dr. Chen has lived or to which he has traveled as a public health physician. Emphasis is given to the organization, at Dingxian, of the first systematic rural health system in the nation and to the lessons drawn from that experience that may apply to the needs of village populations throughout the world today, including those of China. Dr. Chen also examines other topics on the basis of his own firsthand observation: relations between traditional and modern medicine, the quality of rural health manpower, and trends in medical and public health education.

By the same token, readers interested in subjects that are outside

Dr. Chen's direct sphere of interest and activity may find their expectations unfulfilled. For examples, some readers may be disappointed that the account gives relatively little attention to family planning in China, a subject that arouses considerable interest in foreign observers. Family planning, however, is not one of the author's own areas of interest or specialization. Moreover, its policy and planning aspects are the responsibility of an agency other than the Ministry of Health, of whose activities Dr. Chen has no direct knowledge.

While Dr. Chen furnished basic layouts for the two maps in the study, the final versions and the two other figures were prepared in Washington, D.C. by a professional graphic artist and cartographer and former colleague, Harriett R. Blood. Again, if these illustrations contain any errors or omissions, the responsibility is mine alone. Denise D. Grant, also of Washington D.C., whom I came to know through the course of this study, very kindly lent selected private papers of John B. Grant used in the preparation of chapters 2 and 3.

It has been an honor to work with Dr. Chen, whom I, like countless others, hold in the highest respect. His work, I believe, is one of great importance and should contribute in an absolutely critical way to the furtherance of community medicine among rural populations throughout the world.

Berkeley, California   Frederica M. Bunge
December 1987

Acknowledgments

I am indebted to the Health Science Division of the Rockefeller Foundation for a generous grant, which made it possible for me to escape from routine duties in China and to sit down quietly on the beautiful Berkeley campus of the University of California to think and write.

So many friends have extended assistance and suggestions during the course of this work that I can thank them all only by a general reference. I am especially grateful to Professor Peter Kong-Min New and to my brother, Professor Jerome Chen, who read and revised my original draft with respect to both content and language, and to Henrik L. Blum, M.D. of the School of Public Health at the University of California, Berkeley.

I wanted particularly, however, to thank Joyce C. Lashof, M.D., Dean and Professor of Public Health at the School of Public Health in Berkeley, and Kerr L. White, M.D. of the Rockefeller Foundation for their efforts to facilitate my visit to the United States and to provide support and assistance for the work. I am especially grateful for their persistence in securing the necessary provisions for the realization of a personal desire and responsibility to all those who have educated and helped me in over a half a century of my career.

Introduction

$\mathbf{A}$s a scientifically trained physician, I have devoted more than five decades to the work of diffusing modern medicine in rural China, where over 80 percent of our population is to be found. The search for the best means of doing so has been the central concern of my life and provides the central thesis of these memoirs.

My interest in extending the benefits of modern health care to China's hundreds of millions of villagers stems from several strongly held beliefs, namely, that the strength of any nation lies in its common people; that the benefits offered by scientific medicine, introduced from the West, surpass those of our own traditional medicine in most respects; and that a significant impact on the national health system is produced only when the benefits of modern medicine are made available to the general population, rather than limited to a privileged few.

As a consequence of these beliefs, I have devoted my life to the development of community medicine in China. Community medicine, as I perceive it, is a scientific approach to health care based on the needs and conditions of entire populations, rather than on those of individuals alone, and on combining curative and preventive approaches, rather than relying on curative techniques alone. As I define it, it includes epidemiology, vital statistics, and health administration. It represents a more advanced approach to health care than does individualized medicine, a simple relationship between physician and patient.

The basic premises of my medical philosophy, which were established many years ago—deriving from my personal experiences as a child and as a young medical student—have provided a steadying influence, giving purpose and direction through the twists and turns of a life that has followed a rather tortuous course.

My life began, at the turn of the century, as that of an underprivileged child, in an old-style scholar's family in a remote region of China. Because of the insular environment and the unavailability of formal schooling until I reached the age of ten, my early awareness of the outside world was very slight. Offsetting this lack of sophistication, however, was the exposure, given me by my grandfather, to the rich legacy of thought underlying China's age-old civilization.

The inspiration for a life centered on improving the general welfare derived from that formative exposure to our history and culture. Confucian tradition taught that scholars are a special class, but that, with this respected status, went the responsibility, as educated men, of working for the good of the common people. An ancient Chinese teaching, roughly translated, asserts: "People are the foundation of a nation. When the foundation becomes firm, the nation becomes stabilized."

This concept, I believe, captures a principle of long standing in Chinese social philosophy, one that has influenced not only myself but countless generations of Chinese youth educated in our age-old intellectual traditions. It was, I suspect, the wellspring for the intense patriotism and political protest that surfaced in the nineteenth century, when China suffered a painful sequence of foreign invasions and military defeats. More recently, in modern times, concern for the nation and the well-being of the common people has imparted urgency to efforts for social reform and modernization. Developing countries that lack this tradition, I expect, must strive especially hard to develop leaders willing to sacrifice their personal ambitions for the sake of the general welfare.

To return to formative experiences in my life, probably the most consequential were the eight years spent as a young medical student at the Rockefeller Foundation-sponsored Peking Union Medical College (PUMC) in Beijing during the 1920s. There, in that center of academic excellence, I received an education in science and scientific medicine that was of lasting importance to me. It left no question in my mind of the superiority of modern medicine to our own traditional system, nor any doubt of its potential value for improving our national health, provided the people understood its principles correctly.

At the PUMC I met John B. Grant, M.D., whose influence, first as a teacher, and later as a counselor and a friend, was enduring. Grant introduced me to the concept of community medicine and led me to recognize the hazards involved in adopting foreign models in toto, rather than adapting medical practice to local needs and conditions. Equally important, he guided me toward a public health career, arguing that in so doing I could make a far more significant contribution to China than by specializing in dermatology.

As is well known, our country has undergone sweeping social and political change during the past century and a half. The millennia-old Chinese empire disintegrated in 1911, and for several decades thereafter, China suffered fragmentation and internal strife as rival groups struggled for power. Liberation in 1949, however, brought unity and stability once again under the undisputed leadership of the Chinese Communist party (CCP) and paved the way for fundamentally new forms of political, economic, and social institutions and behavior. In furthering the revolution on the scientific and technical fronts, the CCP leadership has sometimes sought, and sometimes avoided, exchange with the outside world.

The Chinese experience in rural health development was considerably affected, both beneficially and adversely by events that unfolded against this backdrop of history. More than a century ago, Western missionaries introduced scientific medicine into our country, with all its potential for improving public health, and over the next century they established scores upon scores of modern hospitals and clinics in Chinese cities. Their efforts benefited a small segment of the population but established a pattern of individualized medicine that focused on curative treatment. This pattern was difficult to eradicate.

Meanwhile, in the 1920s, modern physicians, including Chinese nationals, inadvertently delayed the diffusion of scientific medicine probably by many decades through their demands for the abolition of traditional medicine. Fear generated by their actions caused a powerful coterie of traditional scholar-physicians in the cities to organize for collective action and to seek the intervention of high officials on their behalf. Respected by officials and the public alike, the scholar-physicians were able not only to defend what they already had but also to further extend their influence. More than fifty years later, the two systems of medicine stood on equal footing in China, each with its own schools, treatment facilities, and highly placed friends in the bureaucracy.

The Chinese health experience was also significantly influenced by the Soviet model of public health teaching after 1949 and the expansion of the rural health care infrastructure after 1958. The expansion of rural health services occurred on a scale that few might have believed possible in so short a time and was a remarkable achievement.

The solution of one problem often sets the stage for the emergence of another, however, and in this case many rural health personnel drawn into the system at that time were insufficiently trained to ensure high-quality health care in rural areas. By the mid-1980s their requirements for further training had become an issue of considerable importance.

Personal experience has taught me a great deal over this long period, and in the final chapter of these memoirs, I have tried to share insights from lessons learned. In sum, I believe that we have made memorable strides in extending health care to the common people of China. No part of our country today is without access to modern medicine, and mortality rates have been significantly lowered through mass immunizations against infectious disease. Further health benefits will derive, I believe, from any momentum we can add to a shift from hospital- and clinic-based individualized medicine to population-based medicine, combining curative and preventive approaches.

Efforts to upgrade and develop consistent standards in the training of local health personnel and to recruit medical students who are public health-minded will add to the well-being of the people. As of 1987, there was enormous variation in the depth and length of training of our rural health personnel. Improvement of quality will be realized only through the further education of these personnel. The strengthening of undergraduate medical education in public health should be given priority, with additional emphasis on fieldwork. Problem-solving specialists in public health will be most effective when rural health personnel have had a sound, well-rounded academic background before beginning their specialized training.

Experience provides other insights as well. For example, it indicates the need to support experimentation directed at finding solutions appropriate to local needs and conditions and developing innovative and idealistic leadership. Continuous progress requires constant professional exchange and, in many cases, foreign assistance.

Also in China, where scientific medicine exists side by side with a deeply entrenched and politically endorsed indigenous system of medicine, it may be particularly important that modern-trained physicians maintain the highest possible standards of practice. When scientifically trained physicians make mistakes in diagnosis, for example, popular confidence in scientific medicine is diminished and its diffusion in society is decelerated.

In writing these memoirs, I recall that Confucius stated that "at the age of fifty one realizes what fate heaven has bestowed on him." Life expectancy has increased greatly over the millenia since Confucius lived. In present-day China a person of fifty can still look forward to what may be the crowning lifetime achievement. Even one several decades older than that can still envision ways in which he can contribute to making one's nation stronger, one's people better off.

Naturally, though, any thinking person who has already lived over eighty years, as I have, is inclined to ponder more over present and past personal achievements than future personal plans and objectives. And, in that context, most of us are apt to be surprised to realize how little we have accomplished in our lifetimes. We might have thought a lot about others; however, in terms of what we actually have been able to do to improve the well-being of others, failures usually outnumber successes.

What the eventual impact of my own work may be, perhaps only time will tell. Over the course of my lifetime, my professional influence has waxed and waned. In the mid-1980s, respect for my work was continuing to grow, and I can only hope that in time it will contribute to some degree to the social welfare of our common people, to whom I am devoted. Whatever the case, I am glad that despite many ups and downs, I have been able to keep to my original intention to serve the people.

The problems that I have faced are universal. Perhaps very few other physicians, however, have considered them over as long a period as the fifty-plus working years through which I have passed. Some physicians may have had less contact with indigenous medicine than I; others may not have lived in a period when social conditions stimulated patriotism and participation in the work of awakening the public in health matters. Some may not have had the chance of experimenting on a health system to reach the villagers. Others may not have lived in both capitalistic and socialist societies. Still others may not have had so much to do with educational work of different types as I have. Thus, my varied personal experiences may be of interest to quite a cross section of health workers. Those who have faced similar problems may learn something, while others may find my experience irrelevant. Perhaps one inference that can be justifiably drawn from these reflections on my life in the context of rural health development in China is that it may take people a long time to realize the significance of any new, progressive, and far-reaching idea.

Community-oriented physicians are badly needed. Numerous experiences show that an integrated health delivery system, with dedicated administrators and an enthusiastic,—if only minimally trained—village-level staff, can indeed gradually bring the benefits of scientific medical knowledge to the villagers. The fundamental approach to a human endeavor of lasting value must be through education in various forms. Only when the villagers are touched with the rudiments of health information and techniques will there be hope for "health for all by the year 2000."

PART I

Preliberation China

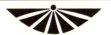

Encounter Between Two Medicines

As a child in the city of Chengdu, China in the early 1900s, I often heard people striking gongs in our neighborhood. Sometimes I would go to take a look, finding that someone was ill, usually lying in bed. The sound of gongs, together with the smell of burning incense, was supposed to drive away ghosts believed to be haunting the sick. I dimly remember that this kind of incantation has been rendered in our home—consisting of three dark rooms—during my mother's final illness. What that ritual was all about, I had no idea. I only knew that it had not saved my mother, and that she had died of some unknown disease.

The circumstances of the deaths of my mother and later my stepmother left me determined to alleviate the cycle of illness, suffering, and death besetting my family. I had seen that disease was terrible, and that indigenous Chinese medicine, formulated by respected Confucian scholars and endorsed by high-ranking officials and the emperors, had nonetheless been useless in eradicating this disease. Even as a boy, therefore, I was already convinced that our traditional methods of dealing with disease was inadequate, and that other methods must be found.

Like most Chinese, young or old, I was unaware at the time that modern medicine even existed. Imperial policies had kept China in seclusion for centuries. Science and scientific thinking as it evolved in the West had made significant inroads only in the nineteenth century, and even then the impact was confined largely to the so-

called treaty ports and other coastal cities, where foreign diplo-
mats, business executives, missionaries, and educators plied their
trades.

To be sure, "Western," or "modern," medicine had been introduced into Guangzhou (Canton), Shanghai, and other cities more
than half a century before my birth. This development, however,
had little or no meaning for most Chinese. For the empire's citizenry
at that time was both vast—numbering well over 400 million—and
overwhelmingly rural.[1] The peasantry, moreover, was scattered
over an enormous expanse of territory in a myriad of tiny villages
and small towns that were linked only by the most rudimentary
channels of transport and communication. Among the common people, literacy was rare and news traveled slowly.

Chengdu, where I had been born and had spent my childhood,
lay in interior China, about 1,000 miles southwest of Shanghai. Its
inhabitants neither knew of, nor had access to, modern medical
care. In sickness and suffering, they depended for help solely on
indigenous Chinese medicine—a set of beliefs and practices that
had been handed down over the ages and was deeply rooted in
the Confucian-based cultural tradition that governed their daily
lives. They trusted in it, for its worth had been vouchsafed by
classical scholars and emperors and tested over countless previous generations.

Confident in this endorsement, the people of Chengdu and surrounding villages trusted traditional medicine and seldom, if ever,
questioned its value—regardless of evident shortcomings. In this,
they mirrored the behavior of other persons throughout rural
China.

THE LATE IMPERIAL PERIOD TO 1911

The limited diffusion of modern, or scientific, medicine in the
China I knew as a child reflected the long-time imperial policy of
global isolation. This policy had deprived China of the benefits of
scientific discovery and industrialization over an extended period.

The attitude that foreign goods and ideas were neither needed
nor wanted had evolved during the two and one-half centuries of
stability under Ming rule (1368–1644) and persisted through the
first two centuries of Qing rule (1644–1911) under alien Manchu

overlords.[2] During the Ming and Qing dynasties, economy, art, and society had flourished.

Comparison of China's achievements in these fields with those of the less developed peoples along its land borders gave rise to the view among Chinese that their empire was the self-sufficient center of the universe. The cultural superiority of Chinese civilization had seemed indisputable. To protect this unique and cherished legacy from despoilation by foreigners, therefore, a succession of emperors had opted for safety in seclusion. As a result, over many centuries China developed as an inward-oriented, backward-looking society.[3]

The history of the high cost of this policy is well known. Chinese civilization had, indeed, enjoyed many years of stability, growth, and prosperity. Meanwhile, however, its classical Confucian scholars remained unenlightened as to the intellectual and scientific advances made in Europe during and after the Industrial Revolution. Bypassed in this way, the Chinese empire fell far behind the West in scientific and technological spheres.[4]

In the nineteenth century, the imperial government found itself gravely threatened by foreign military forces and unprepared to deal with them. A series of engagements with foreign troops armed with vastly superior weaponry inflicted defeats that the Chinese people felt as deeply humiliating. The image of the emperor and his retinue was severely damaged by these happenings, and their domestic support base was further eroded by economic difficulties, which led to widespread peasant revolts.

The dissolution of power had begun with the military defeat delivered by the British during the first Opium War (1839–1842), during the aftermath of which China was compelled to make major trade and territorial concessions to Western nations. Anti-Manchu sentiment escalated in the countryside, reflected in various plots and revolts, including the thirteen-year Taiping Rebellion (1851–1864).[5]

Droughts, flood, and famine, disrupting economic production, brought suffering to many villagers, who depended on farming for their livelihoods. Although the villagers constituted the economic backbone of the nation, the imperial government assumed little responsibility for prevention, or alleviation, of such disasters.[6] In life-and-death matters, the people relied on each other, and on what help they could get from practitioners of traditional medicine.

With public health planning and policy nonexistent, disease was commonplace and intermittent epidemics caused many deaths.

While doing little to aid the villagers, the government in the 1860s instituted—if reluctantly—certain "self-strengthening" reforms that resulted in a modicum of industrial development. Shipyards, arsenals, and textile mills were added in places to the urban landscape.[7] A few foreign language and technical schools were opened under official auspices. The government supported translation of a number of foreign scientific and technical publications. In all, however, the impact of the reforms was modest. They barely touched rural China.

The situation changed significantly after China's defeat by Japan in Korea (1894/95).[8] In the final decade before its collapse, the imperial government, hoping to reassert its authority by whatever means, instituted some important reforms, including educational and military modernization along Japanese lines. Students, sent mainly at government expense, flocked to universities abroad to expose themselves to Western learning and scientific thinking.

The belated reforms were too little and too late. Opposition gathered under republican and anti-Manchu activist Sun Yat-sen, and in October 1911, revolution broke out in South China, spreading over most of the country. On January 1, 1912, the republic of China was proclaimed, signaling the end of 2,000 years of dynastic rule.[9]

TRADITIONAL MEDICINE, EVOLUTION AND ENTRENCHMENT

Our indigenous medicine developed over a period spanning thousands of years, embedding itself in the culture as it evolved. Historians discern three overlapping stages in the process: sorcery, experimentation (mainly with herbs), and classical study and prescription.

STAGES OF DEVELOPMENT

Primitive medicine practiced in ancient times was associated with witches and sorcerers. While society despised such persons, it nonetheless relied on them heavily, for they dominated the art of healing. Their methods, based on superstition, featured supplication to many gods and banishment of evil spirits. In the next stage, beginning with the Shang period, from about 1500 to 1100 B.C, superstitious practices were gradually replaced by remedies sought from nature. Familiar with plant life, villagers looking for sources of relief from illness began to experiment with local flora and fauna. They tried grass, wood, stone, cereals, and insects, all chosen according to their shape, color, smell, and taste.[10]

Through trial and error, an increasing number of herbs were gradually identified as suitable for use, notwithstanding the intoxication that sometimes resulted from excessive dosage. Certain villagers began to specialize in collecting, preparing, and selling them, and if the patient recovered, the herb vendor and the vendor's prescription were usually given credit.

During the Chou period (sometimes dated from 1122 to 221 B.C.), as feudal rulers began to search for safe drugs for themselves, faith in witchcraft declined and respect for herbal medicine increased. Practitioners of herbal medicine were not despised, as the witches had been, but medical practice was still regarded as a somewhat dubious undertaking, and herb vendors were far from being esteemed persons. Most were, in fact, illiterate. Their lowly status was evident in a disparaging remark attributed to Confucius: "Without perseverance or hard work, one could not even become a doctor or a witch." A popular saying admonished, too, that "only medicine offered by practitioners after three generations of family practice can be trusted."

Indigenous medicine entered its third stage of development, after much of what came to constitute China Proper was unified for the first time in 221 B.C. Qin (Ch'in) emperors began to enlist scholars to study medicine and to attempt to develop theories that explained various diseases and their origins. These scholars had extensive knowledge of philosophy and other aspects of classical learning, according to which they could interpret human and social phenomena. Eventually they worked out medical classics, based in part on these sources.

For example, *yin/yang* theory had constituted an important strain of thought in Chinese philosophy since the Eastern Zhou (Chou) period 771–221 B.C. Yin/yang theory essentially held that all cosmic forces are composed of mutually complementary opposites: *yang*—sun, light, hot, male, and positive; *yin*—moon, dark, cold, female, and negative.[11] This dualism had long been useful in explaining many phenomena in the universe, and scholar-physicians were able to correlate their ideas regarding the etiology of disease, diagnosis, and in certain instances treatment, with its postulates.

Working out their ideas in this way, through a combination of their own experience and an analysis of classical literature, the scholar-physicians (*ru-yi*) were able to offer theoretical explanations of medical phenomena that scholars in other fields accepted as legitimate. The two groups spoke from a basis of common understanding in language and learning. Equally important, the explanations of the scholar-physicians were credible to ordinary Chinese because they were consistent with what people had already accepted on faith as part of their cultural tradition.

In the unity and prosperity of the Han period (206 B.C.–A.D. 220) medicine made unprecedented strides, and scholar-physicians solidified their new exalted position at the court. Emperor Wu-di coined the title "Scholar of Prescriptions" for the scholar-physicians who served the court. Emperor He-di established an imperial medical bureau—the first government medical organization, and appointed Guoyu, a highly respected scholar, as its chief. Imperial physicians began to feel that the pulse was an index for the objective detection of ill health. They developed acupuncture, a medical technique based on a traditional Taoist theory that maintenance of health depends on free circulation of *T'chi* (life-force energy, controlled by yin/yang balance). One of the best known acupuncture practitioners was Hua Tuo (A.D. 110–207), who also performed surgical operations under alcohol-induced anesthesia and, stressing prevention, emphasized the importance of physical exercise in health promotion and maintenance. He encouraged people to imitate the bird, monkey, deer, bear, tiger, and horse in motion. He indicated that the limbs and torso could become supple and strong, blood could circulate regularly, and diseases of the extremities could be prevented.

The scholar-physicians of the Jin (Chin) dynasty (A.D. 265–420) contributed significantly to the formulation of medical classics, collectively producing 256 medical treatises. Their broad-based knowledge rarely benefited the general public, however, as they served chiefly the emperor and court officials. Practitioners dealing with the needs of the general public relied for the most part on a single reference work, *Zhou Hou Fang*. The emperor rarely, if ever, personally assumed responsibility for unmet health needs.

Despite the gratifying nature of their new position, some scholar-physicians were uncomfortably aware of the shortcomings of medical practice at that time. One wrote: "The practitioners of today merely inherit ideas from their predecessors and prescribe drugs without much thought; they are quite unable to cure difficult cases."

In the millennium between the start of the Song dynasty (A.D. 960–1279) and the close of the imperial period in 1911, Chinese society wholly embraced indigenous medicine. In various periods, medical institutions were established to serve the imperial household, to regulate medical practice, and to stimulate medical thought. For example, the Song emperors founded an imperial medical college whose scholars ultimately produced an extensive body of medical literature. Yuan rulers (A.D. 1279–1368) organized an imperial college of physicians. The reputation of Chinese medicine spread to Japan, and during two centuries of Ming rule, a number of Japanese medical students were permitted to come to China to gain an appreciation of Chinese medical principles.

Death and morbidity rates from communicable and infectious diseases were extremely high. Few Chinese at the time accepted the general concept that the environment influences the incidence of disease, or that many diseases are contagious; thus, prevention was given little consideration. Curative, rather than preventive, medicine was seen as the essential component of health care.

Scholar-physicians served the wealthy elite of urban China; undereducated and largely self-taught traditional practitioners provided medical relief for other urban dwellers and to rural China. In both cases, herbalists represented the majority of practitioners; demand for their services far exceeded that for acupuncturists and surgeons.

Qing officialdom assumed no responsibility for oversight of the medical field. Medical education was informal and practice was wholly unregulated. It was a free-for-all. Much of what transpired between patient and physician, moreover, was enveloped in an aura of secrecy. Sharing of experience among practitioners was uncommon. In fact, successful treatments were often kept from the knowledge of competing physicians.

CONSOLIDATION OF THE POSITION OF
TRADITIONAL MEDICINE

If indigenous medicine had been left entirely in the hands of village practitioners and if its approach to treatment had continued to be based on superstition and empirical experience alone, public confidence in it would probably have gradually declined. In rural areas traditional practitioners were typically no different from their urban counterparts. They were simple, peasant farmers, unable to read and write. What they knew about healing arts had been self-taught or learned through apprenticeship. Herbal remedies and superstitious practices were all they could recommend for medical relief.

Once imperial interest had focused the attention of urban-based classical scholars on the study of medicine, however, the perpetuity of traditional medicine was assured. Scholar-officials turned to ancient Chinese classics for insight, assembling a body of literature to validate the methods of treatment that were thereafter applied. Later generations of scholar-physicians (a subclass of scholar-officials), concentrated in the cities, had access to a growing library of medical texts and learned through empirical trials as well as through reading and study. The substance of traditional medicine as practiced in urban China eventually differed quite markedly from its rural variant. In many cases treatment was very likely more efficacious, and in any event, patient confidence in this form of traditional practice was reinforced by prevailing respect for ancient classical learning. In the process, the principles of medicine formulated by the scholar-physicians were legitimized by ancient classical thought, and in time, an attack on traditional medicine came to be regarded as an attack on the cherished national cultural heritage itself.

The perpetuation of traditional medicine was further assured by the broadening political base of this form of medical practice. Over the centuries, quite naturally, scholar-physicians developed a vested interest in the viability of their vocation, while, in their professional capacity, they acquired high social standing and important connections. As educated men, they had many friends in high places. They spoke the same language and shared the same background as scholar-officials. In fact, some were scholar-officials themselves or were related to them through kinship ties. By 1911 scholar-physicians had so solidified their position that traditional medicine not only survived the collapse of the old feudal order under which it had become so entrenched but also expanded and prospered. Persons interested in health and medical in China today would learn a great deal by studying that entrenchment process.

CHRISTIAN MISSIONARIES AND THE ADVENT OF MODERN MEDICINE

Modern, or scientific, medicine, introduced by Christian missionaries from the West, mainly the United States, initially offered little or no challenge to the preeminence of traditional medicine. Although some work was done in outlying rural centers, missionary medical practice was confined largely to urban hospitals and clinics. Then, as now, however, only a small minority of Chinese lived in the cities, and the patient load of even these urban facilities was small relative to the total urban population. As for the rural majority, it had almost no knowledge of, or experience with, modern medicine whatsoever.

Limited penetration was not the only reason for the relative unimportance of scientific medicine as of 1911. Modern medicine had evolved out of an alien civilization, with whose institutions and patterns of behavior it was difficult for the Chinese to identify. Modern medicine had been borrowed whole, in no way adapted to fit Chinese resources or conditions. It was part of a foreign way of thinking, in an era when foreign ideas were highly suspect or unwelcome. Traditional medicine, by contrast, was anchored in the Chinese world view and was suited to Chinese-perceived realities.

MISSIONARY MEDICINE

Missionary medical activity began in China in the early 1830s but rapidly expanded in the latter part of the nineteenth century, seemingly as sponsors in the West became convinced of its potential as a channel for Christian proselytization. Medical work by missionary physicians was generally associated with the dissemination of Christian beliefs and the message of conversion, although the paramountcy of the medical versus the evangelical goal varied from time to time and place to place.[12]

The first missionary fully trained as a physician was Peter Parker, who established a clinic in Guangzhou in 1835. There, despite his unfamiliarity with antisepsis or anesthesia, Parker treated a variety of simple ailments and performed various surgical procedures with a degree of success that won him many patients.[13] That small beginning heralded what in the late nineteenth century became a substantial medical missionary effort, as sponsors in the United States and Canada grew increasingly enthusiastic about evangelist prospects. A Western chronicle notes that the number of missionary hospitals increased from 10 to 61 between 1850 and 1889, and that within another fifteen years or so the number of missionary hospitals had risen to 362. In addition, there were 244 ambulatory-care facilities.[14]

Missionaries also established many teaching hospitals and medical colleges as well, including Hunan-Yale Medical College in Changsha, Hunan Province; Saint John's College in Shanghai; Lingnan University in Guangzhou; Union Medical College in Beijing; and West China Union University schools of dentistry and medicine in Chengdu, Sichuan Province. There was also a French-sponsored Roman Catholic school in Shanghai. In addition to the missionary schools, there was a German medical college under secular administration.

The content and method of teaching in these institutions were patterned mainly on the basis of Anglo-American models. After completing what in most cases was a six-year curriculum, graduates usually went to work in a missionary hospital or entered private practice.

This was consistent with the basic missionary approach to health care, in which the central frame of reference was the hospital or the clinic, providing treatment for individual patients. Missionaries began by building facilities for patient care, and although they undertook some immunization efforts and did some health education work, their main thrust while in China was on curative medicine.

Returned Students

Meanwhile, among the urban educated elite, many young persons were beginning to see that their ambitions might be just as well satisfied by studying modern medicine as by reading the Chinese classics in the hope of becoming scholar-officials. Some enrolled in missionary colleges; however, foreign schools—a few in Britain and the United States, but especially those in Japan—drew larger numbers. By 1910 the number of students, including medical students, enrolled in Western institutions exceeded 10,000. After returning home, those who had studied abroad were commonly referred to as "returned students."[15]

Graduates in medicine among this foreign-educated group were interested in keeping abreast of developments in their field through contact and discussion with other modern physicians. A logical forum would have been the medical association that missionary physicians had organized and to which many belonged, notwithstanding the fact that the functions of that group had become largely social. To their disillusionment, however, the returned students found themselves barred from membership in the missionary organization. Accordingly, in 1915 they founded their own group, which in time absorbed the missionary-established group.

Relations with Scholar-Physicians

At that time relations between the two groups of Chinese physicians—modern and traditional—were no more productive or extensive than those between the two groups of modern physicians. In fact, like missionary physicians, modern Chinese physicians were generally disdainful of traditional medicine, displaying little respect for it as a discipline or for its practitioners as individuals. For the most part, their attitude was nonchalant at best and at times frankly contemptuous.

Centuries of trial and error had produced a large body of experience as well as a pharmacopoeia that warranted at least some degree of scientific investigation. Yet returned students and medical missionaries paid no attention to it. Quite to the contrary, they ignored any possibilities for collaboration in either research or practice. Modern physicians were totally complacent in their belief in the superiority of European achievement in medicine, and the merits or demerits of traditional medicine were a matter of indifference to them.

One or two modern medical scientists were exceptions to the prevailing attitude, expressing respect for traditional practitioners and acknowledging that some traditional remedies might be worthy of scientific observation. One of these persons was Dr. Edward H. Hume, a medical missionary at Hunan–Yale Medical College. Another was Wu Lien-teh, a returned student from Britain and a modern physician of national stature. Wu's positive attitude toward traditional medicine was particularly significant, insofar as it had been he who, through the use of a scientifically based immunization campaign, had finally contained a nation-threatening plague outbreak in Manchuria, against which traditional practitioners had been totally helpless.

In fact, containment of the Manchurian plague by means of a massive scientifically based immunization campaign had been a watershed event in the history of modern medicine in our country, disposing many Chinese more favorably to a system previously rejected for its foreign origin. Wu's success in halting the tide of death was to many persons a telling demonstration of the value of scientific procedures. Government officials, ordinary people, and even some traditional practitioners came to see this medicine from the West in a new light, thinking it might after all have some value for China.

Aside from this episode, however, traditional scholar-physicians in those days were as unimpressed by modern physicians as modern physicians were by them. Far from feeling themselves threatened by the new medicine from the West, they knew the extent of their support and recognized that most Chinese regarded modern medicine as "foreign" and not to be trusted except perhaps with respect to surgery. At that time, it was commonplace to hear someone assert that missionary physicians and Western medicine were competent in surgical cases, but that one should still rely on indigenous medicine for treatment of disease. This attitude was understandable for the groundwork for a generalized appreciation of science, and scientific principles had not yet been laid in our country.

A LIFETIME RESOLVE TAKES SHAPE

Chengdu, of course, was far away from China's capital, Beijing, where a minority of persons were coming to regard science and scientific thinking as a force that could bring great benefit to our society. It was far, too, from Manchuria, where Wu had so dramatically demonstrated the efficacy of modern medical procedures. Word—even of climactic events in other parts of the empire—reached us belatedly, if at all.

In that isolated part of China (highways and rail transportation came only much later) we were dependent on ourselves and on traditional resources. When herbal remedies failed, we occasionally even resorted to practices based on superstition. For example, when I was twelve years of age, I contracted malaria, for which there was no effective treatment. In a desperate attempt to save my life, however, my family subjected me to having my legs whipped and forced me to run around in a courtyard with firecrackers exploding under my knees. The hope was that the noise would drive away the evil spirits that might be causing my illness.

It was not my own experiences, however, but the lingering illnesses and deaths of other family members that made me feel so keenly the need for another way to cope with disease. I had never seen my paternal grandparents; they died very early. After my mother's death, which I learned much later was caused by tuberculosis of the spine, and before my father's remarriage, I had gone to live briefly with my maternal grandparents. My grandfather, who had been educated in the Chinese classics, tutored me at home.

At one time or another, my father's household in Chengdu included, besides myself, my mother, my younger brother, my elder sister, and my father's brother and sister. My uncle disappeared one day, never to be seen again. Like most Chinese youth of his day, he had had no education and, unable to support himself, and being reluctant to add to the burdens of the family, he chose to fade into oblivion. Apart from my father and his brother, everyone in the household died during my childhood. My father's sister, possibly like my mother, succumbed to tuberculosis and my brother, to typhoid fever. What illness took my sister's life we never knew.

My father remarried, and then, just as I was able to attend a formal school for the first time, my stepmother contracted a serious illness. We did not know what she was suffering from at the time, either, although later I was able to deduce that she had contracted pulmonary tuberculosis. Her illness was distressing, as she had been very good to me in many ways, always treating me kindly, and encouraging me to obtain as much education as possible.

Fearing that traditional medicine would fail her, as it had so utterly failed my own mother, I subconsciously vowed to try to find something to help her. Because of this childhood experience with suffering, disease, and death, from an early age I was determined to find another, better system of medicine and to make that medicine available throughout urban and rural China.

2

Ideas and Ideals: Medical Students and Social Change

At the age of fourteen in 1917, I accompanied my stepmother to the French consulate in Chengdu, where she went as a last resort seeking treatment for her illness. The attending physician examined her, using a thermometer, a stethoscope, and, to take her blood pressure, a sphygmomanometer. I was impressed by the status and prestige the physician seemed to enjoy, and more so by the scientific instruments at his disposal. Then and there, I determined to become a modern physician myself. I had no idea how this could be accomplished, of course, and much less any notion that it would require years of formal study.

Nonetheless, aided by a chance event or two, considerable determination, and the boyhood conviction that no dream, however distant, is impossible to fulfill, I managed to achieve my ambition within little more than a decade. In 1921 I was admitted to an elite medical college, newly established in Beijing by an American philanthropic organization, and in 1929 I graduated from that institution as a fully qualified physician. Academic, geographic, and economic obstacles, not to mention a linguistic barrier, had stood in the way of reaching that milestone. Such were the difficulties, however, that confronted many young people who aspired to higher education in our country at that time.

The world that I knew as a student at the Peking Union Medical College (PUMC) from 1921 to 1929 was far removed from that of my boyhood in Chengdu. I had exchanged the isolated intellectual realm of traditional society for the expansive world of science and scientific thinking. Beijing in North China was a huge city, pulsating with life. It was China's capital and the 1920s was a turbulent era of growing national consciousness, as recurrent antiimperialist and antigovernment protest merged with reformist intellectual currents to forge a national cultural awakening.

Intellectuals and students were calling for wholesale national renewal, and, in that process, science was seen to be the key. In fact, to many influential persons in public life, the potentialities of science and scientific thinking for the betterment of human life seemed almost boundless. Science became, in effect, a philosophical doctrine whose precepts could be applied to issues and problems in all realms of life.

At the PUMC I was deeply absorbed in my scientific studies. Nonetheless, beginning in 1925, I became increasingly caught up in the fervor of the national awakening and engrossed in the academic and social issues it engendered. My intensifying patriotism made me more determined than ever to find some way to improve the health of our common people. The appeals of science and social conscience were competing for my time and attention.

Resolution of this dilemma came after I began public health studies in 1926 under John B. Grant, M.D. Grant, the Far Eastern representative of the International Health Divison of the Rockefeller Foundation, had been detailed to establish a department of public health at the college. Grant was concerned with the whole spectrum of social medicine, and unlike many of his peers, was less interested in the pursuit of scientific knowledge for its own sake than for its applications for the betterment of human life. His medical philosophy was multifaceted, emphasizing community-based planning and a combination of curative and preventive services.

To this end, he constantly focused the attention of students on conditions in their own country, choosing lecture material that was relevant for China. He always illustrated his points with local or regional examples and arranged for training outside the classroom to provide us with firsthand exposure to real-life situations. For many students, the face-to-face exposure to the suffering of clinical patients and their increasing awareness of the health problems of millions of Chinese men, women, and children in the countryside was a shocking experience. It was true, as Grant had noted, that poor health was in part responsible for China's weakness.

As we delved more and more deeply into public health studies, the critical relationship of public health to national renewal became increasingly clear. We saw public health promotion as an urgent issue, especially with respect to prevention. Private practice, however attractive, would not contribute much to society. In time several classmates and I decided to forego its rewards and devote ourselves instead to pioneering in the development of a health system to meet the needs of rural people.

On hearing Grant insist on the adaptation of practice to the realities of China, I reached a critical realization: rather than rely on a borrowed medical school model in our efforts to bring modern medicine to the people, China must create a new model, based on its own conditions and its own resources. Foreign models were fraught with risks and problems. That insight has remained with me throughout my life.

The issue then became how we could best introduce modern scientific medicine into a predominantly rural population and make it take root there for the benefit of the entire country. I have been concerned with this issue ever since I left medical school.

PRELIBERATION CHINA: 1912 to 1928

For most of the years I spent as a student in Beijing, the city was the internationally recognized capital of the Chinese Republic. China, however, was unable to achieve even nominal unity until 1928, and Beijing, meanwhile, was controlled by a succession of warlord regimes. The country itself was beset by civil strife and contending political-military forces in a prolonged crisis of power.[1]

THE HEALTH AND MEDICAL SETTING

Comprehensive and reliable health data for the period 1912–1928 are unavailable because the warlords took no interest in public health, much less in the collection of vital statistics. A country the size of China could not be considered as one unit, and health conditions, of course, varied from place to place. Surveys of Beijing, Shanghai, and Harbin, in Manchuria, nevertheless confirmed the general impression of widespread medical problems.

It was safe to assume that the crude death rate probably exceeded 30 per 1,000; the infant mortality rate was probably about 200 per 1,000 live births; and life expectancy was probably about thirty-five years. Maternal mortality may have exceeded 20 per 1,000, especially in rural areas. Tetanus neonatorum was the number one cause of infant death. It was reported, for example, that in one of the twenty counties included in the municipality of Beijing, many children under one week of age died from tetanus, which at that time had been entirely eradicated from many Western countries. In fact, one village reported that, over the previous ten years, 60 percent of its live-born children had died.[2] Infectious diseases, mostly preventable, accounted for one-third to one-half of all deaths. The birth rate was very high, and numbers of children suffered from various physical defects for which no treatment facilities existed. Intermittent famines caused considerable suffering.

In the mid-1920s there was, to all intents and purposes, no public health organization at the national, provincial, or municipal level. The health-related activities that did take place were conducted under the aegis of the Ministry of the Interior by police authorities. Such measures were few and far between, however, and as the chief of police was a returned student from Germany, German and Japanese models were emulated. They focused mainly on street cleaning, and even that was poorly done.

The single noteworthy government initiative in the health sphere during this period was the establishment in 1919 of a Central Epidemic Prevention Bureau. This move followed in the aftermath of an outbreak of plague in Manchuria that had taken 60,000 lives and an epidemic of pneumonic plague in Suiyuan in northwestern China in 1917. The agency produced some vaccine, mainly for smallpox. Regrettably, however, not long after its establishment, popular concern about disease abated, and most people lost interest in being immunized.

British-trained Wu Lien-teh, who directed the immunization activities in Manchuria, and a few other modern Chinese physicians, were convinced that prevention warranted more emphasis. As early as 1915, at the first meeting of the newly formed "returned student" group, the National Medical Association of China (NMAC), he and Yen Fu-ching had organized a public health committee. They also sponsored a motion making health education an NMAC goal. Wu and Yen also supported a subsequent NMAC recommendation for the formation of a national-level health administration agency and a call for government action against tuberculosis and venereal disease. Wu also attacked the opium problem. At his urging in 1917, the NMAC demanded prohibition of the importation of morphine. Later Wu himself went to Shanghai to destroy 1,200 boxes of imported opium.

Meanwhile, modern scientific medicine had established a strong position in urban China, dominated by medical missionaries whose activites focused on hospitals and clinical treatment. A 1919 missionary report counted 900 Chinese physicians and 600 foreign physicians in China, nearly all in the cities.[3] Medical missionaries were doing some work in rural Hunan Province and a few other outlying areas, but this was an exception to the general urban orientation of missionary medicine.

Modern medical facilities included a few public hospitals and a proliferation of missionary hospitals, medical schools, and dispensaries and one or two private, secularly run institutions. One report estimated the number of missionary hospitals at that time to be well over 300.[4] By far the most prestigious medical institutions, however, were the PUMC and its affiliated hospital. The Rockefeller Foundation had purchased the Union Medical College in Beijing from its missionary founders, and by the early 1920s had developed it into the leading institution in China for the training of physicians and nurses.

Standards in the PUMC hospital were impeccable, but those in many other hospitals were far from satisfactory. One medical missionary association report indicated that the great majority of hospitals lacked a potable water supply and that most had no means of sterilizing beds or mattresses. More than 30 percent lacked laboratory facilities of any kind.[5] Despite these shortcomings, the missionary hospitals provided a large amount of service and in so doing contributed to building a more favorable popular attitude toward modern medicine among the urban population.

Political instability and lack of funds accounted in part for the poor conditions found in public hospitals; however, as important as these were, the low level of scientific awareness was probably still more important. A reporter for the *Binying Weekly*, a newspaper health supplement that several other PUMC students and I had established to raise health consciousness in the capital city, described a visit to a public hospital in Beijing in 1926:

> The curtain at the room's entrance was very dirty; the air was putrid; and the basins at the bedside were filthy. No one seemed to look after the food for the patients, let alone give consideration to nutrition and cleanliness. As the drugs were kept by the patients themselves, there was no assurance they were taken care of properly. All this shows there existed no type of nursing.[6]

As long as the public remained ignorant of the consequences of such unhygienic conditions and unsound medical practices, little would be done to correct the situation.

Given the indifference of the urban population to health hazards, it was hardly surprising to find the situation incomparably worse in rural areas. Indeed, the difference in mentality between urban and rural communities was so great that any scientifically trained physician attempting to work in the countryside faced a formidable task. The relative impoverishment and lack of education of villages produced attitudes, values, and ways of thinking quite at variance with those of urban-born Chinese. The medical students that I knew came mainly from coastal cities and knew little or nothing about the concerns or circumstances of the villagers. In my own case, for instance, I still remember today how strange I found life in a village about ten miles from Chengdu, where I was taken for a visit as a boy of eight.

Two Medicines in Confrontation

Meanwhile, in urban China, intellectual currents emphasizing the application of scientific principles to transform society were being felt in the medical field, as elsewhere. Even traditional medicine was not entirely immune to the effect of these influences. For instance, one Qing dynasty scholar-physician, Wang Qing-ren, attempted to draw some biological inferences from an examination of the visceral organs of children who had died in a measles epidemic, eliciting some interest from a few of his colleagues.

After World War I, the fundamental question posed by Chinese intellectuals regarding Chinese and Western culture and their relative advantages and disadvantages provided the context for a rapidly escalating confrontation between traditional medicine and Western medicine.[7] A number of articles praising "Western medicine" appeared, along with occasional editorials demanding the outright abolition of traditional medicine.

Initially, scholar-physicians showed no great concern over this development, nor did it significantly diminish popular confidence in their modes of treatment. They outnumbered scientifically trained physicians, enjoyed high social status, and shared important political connections.

In 1922, however, the Ministry of the Interior, reacting to pressure from a group of returned students, promulgated a series of regulations governing traditional practice. In view of the freewheeling atmosphere that had prevailed under the Qing dynasty, this was a novel and decidedly unwelcome development for traditional physicians, and it aroused their concern and indignation. Not long afterward, controversy ensued regarding the right of traditional medicine to begin to organize its own formal schools of medicine on a par with modern medical colleges. In addition to this, in 1925 the Chinese Missionary Medical Association demanded that the government prohibit the teaching of modern medicine and that it enforce existing regulations requiring the licensing of traditional practitioners on the basis of a formal examination.

In the face of this onslaught, scholar-physicians organized for collective action, using their connections with the press and links to influential politicians to turn the situation around. Before the year was out, the provinces of Shanxi, Zhejiang, and Hubei had enacted resolutions specifically permitting the establishment and operation of institutions to provide formal instruction in traditional medicine. Further rounds in the struggle were to come.

FROM CHENGDU TO BEIJING: A
STUDENT'S JOURNEY

As the struggle intensified, I was entering adolescence in Chengdu. My stepmother concluded her treatments at the French consulate and I continued to think about becoming a modern physician. My father, an old-style scholar, was sympathetic to this plan but had no more idea than I did how it might be accomplished.

In Chengdu proper, there was a missionary-run modern medical college, the West China Union University, but somehow I had never heard of it. Indirectly, however, I learned of another alternative. An article in the Shanghai press by Li Zhenpian, a male nurse at Hunan–Yale Medical College, attracted my attention. Its author argued the superiority of modern medicine over our own system so thoroughly and convincingly that I decided to contact him, asking him how I could become a student at Hunan–Yale. After a long delay, Li's response arrived. He wrote that an outstanding new medical college had been organized in Beijing, and that it would be a better choice for me than his own school. That was how I first heard of the PUMC.

Gaining Admission to the PUMC

Studying modern medicine was a simple idea, but its realization was no easy matter. Years of preparation were required and thorny problems had to be overcome, not the least of which was cost. Our family's means were quite limited, certainly too restricted to finance my graduate education. Distance was another obstacle. Traveling to Beijing, a thousand miles to the northeast, would be uncommonly difficult, for Chengdu lay in a vast, remote part of southwest China, as yet unconnected by rail or highway to the northern or coastal cities. Most formidable problem of all, however, was the language barrier.

In the missionary medical colleges, instruction was typically offered in Chinese by teachers whose fluency in the language varied from fair to excellent. The PUMC, however, after what seems to have been considerable debate, chose to teach in English, admitting only students who qualified in terms of language capability.

While the PUMC decision was appropriate, it did require a great deal of effort by the candidate and posed enormous difficulty for almost any young Chinese who aspired to study medicine at that time. Some good students were excluded because of the language barrier, and others who circumvented the language requirement initially had to drop out later because their comprehension was inadequate.

In my own case, I began to realize the extent of the problem when a reply to my inquiry regarding admission, written in English arrived at our house in Chengdu. It suggested that, on the basis of the letter I had written, my English was insufficient to enable me to pass the entrance examination.

Not having realized just how inadequate my English was, I was naturally disappointed but became all the more determined to enroll. I found out about and joined a special English class given three times a week by my high-school language instructor, Song Chengzhi, at his church. Song later became an Anglican archdeacon. One of the texts we used was a collection of essays by Ralph Waldo Emerson. As I was doing fairly well, Song later introduced me to a British missionary who agreed to give me private instruction every Sunday. This instruction was concurrent with all my other high-school work.

Acquiring fluency in English was challenge enough in itself, but I soon discovered that to be admitted to the PUMC, I would have to pass English-language entrance examinations in various required subjects, including mathematics, physics, and chemistry. English-language textbooks for these subjects were not available in Chengdu. Few enough young persons studied these subjects in any language, and those who did undertook them in Chinese. After some exploratory correspondence, however, I found a supplier in Shanghai. My stepmother generously gave me funds to buy what was needed. The order took two months to fill, after which time I received a heavy parcel of books. A cousin of my stepmother who knew English and was familiar with scientific terminology offered assistance, and from then on we met every Sunday to work through these textbooks. Until my graduation in the summer of 1921, I studied day and night. Then it was time to try to get to Beijing and pass the admissions tests.

Fortunately for me, a family relative, Mr. Wu, was moving to the capital at that time to work for the government. He had no objection to my accompanying him, and so with my family's approval, we set out, knowing that the trip would be rough and taxing. Sometimes we walked. Sometimes we were carried in a sedan chair. At night we stopped in small hostels, which were invariably dark and dirty. The rooms were illuminated only by small oil lamps similar to the one I had used in high school.

Our first destination was Chongqing, a city larger than Chengdu, lying southeast of it on the Yangtze River. There we boarded a sampan and sailed northeastward through the famous Yangtze River gorges. It was a dangerous voyage, but, as a youth of seventeen, I welcomed the challenge and excitement. Fortunately, we were able to reach Yichang in another ten days, where we changed to a small steamer, somewhat like a modern ferryboat. The boat was crowded, but we managed to find some sleeping space. After four days we reached Hankou in Hubei Province.

Because my traveling companion was exhausted, we rested in Hankou for several days before leaving for Beijing by train, a slow, northward journey of three days. Altogether it had taken us an entire month to cover the 1,000-mile distance between Chengdu and China's capital.

In Beijing, I stayed with the family of a former schoolmate, whose father had become a high official in the Ministry of Education. Eager to see the PUMC, I set off for there on foot at the earliest possible moment. The admissions secretary who had responded to my letter was astonished to see me and to find that I could understand what she said. She endorsed my decision to try entrance examinations.

They were scheduled to be held soon, and I began to prepare at once, moving into a small hostel. The room measured only about six or seven square meters, and a high wall directly opposite the window obstructed the daylight. Not being able to afford an electric reading lamp, I made do with an oil lamp, although this was hard on my eyes. I studied in that dim light, not only all day, but long into the night.

The decisive moment arrived, the first of two successive days of testing. The English-language examination took the entire first morning. We were given text to read from a book no one had ever seen before and were asked to explain its meaning. Dictation followed. The proctor looked for errors in what we had written down. In the afternoon, we were administered an intelligence test—a new concept to me. The time limit was rigid, and I felt a great deal of pressure.

Learning afterward that those who failed would have no further chance, I had difficulty sleeping. The next morning I awoke early and hurried to the school, where I was overjoyed to find my name among those who had passed. This meant that I was eligible to take the tests in Chinese, mathematics, physics, and chemistry, which were to be held that day. After finishing them, we were told to go home.

While awaiting these further results, I continued to study each day, living meanwhile free of charge at the home of a friend of my father, whose hospitality I greatly appreciated. Weeks later I received a notice of acceptance. I was elated, of course, and felt that all the effort of the preceding two years had been worthwhile. It was 1921. I would soon be eighteen years old. A new life was beginning.

PREMEDICAL SCHOOL EXPERIENCES

The living conditions at the PUMC were much better than I had ever had before. An older student, Li Ting-an, who later became the first graduate to take public health as a career, showed me around Lockhart Hall, the old missionary building used as our classroom, and the dormitory behind it. He told me how to make use of all the facilities. I learned that I was the only student from Sichuan Province, in fact the only one from the entire southwestern part of the country. Most of the others were from the coastal cities, mainly Shanghai and Guangzhou.

The caliber of the faculty was high. The PUMC set itself apart from a number of other foreign educational institutions of the day not only in its insistence on English as the language of instruction but also in the distinction of its faculty. This was as true at the premedical school as at the medical school.

All the teachers at the premedical school were competent in their fields, and some went on to achieve academic prominence. Among the latter were physics instructor Dr. W. W. Stifler, later a full professor in physics at a leading university in the United States, and chemistry instructor Dr. S. D. Wilson, later dean of science at Yenching University in Beijing. Other teachers I remember particularly were Dr. Charles W. Packard and Helen R. Downes. Not all the best faculty were foreign, however. There were some particularly well qualified Chinese teaching assistants.

Curriculum requirements during this period compared with those of the best universities in the West. Among other subjects, we studied two foreign languages—English and German, as well as biology, physics, and chemistry. I worked particularly hard on English after the instructor, A. E. Zucker, to my embarrassment once copied out one of my letters on the blackboard so that he could use it to illustrate grammatical errors to the class.

As it was, students took their work very seriously, devoting their time to attending lectures, performing laboratory experiments, reading textbooks, and writing reports, and preparing for examinations, although there were always a few classmates who failed to make the grade. Apart from a glee club and a college publication, *Unison,* and an occasional physical education period, there was little to divert our attention from our main goal, acceptance into the medical school program.

After I passed that critical point in 1924 and was accepted for the medical school program, finances became a real problem. I had won a full-tuition Cochrane Fellowship at the end of the first year of premedical school and had earned my room and board working as a college accountant and dormitory manager. To finance another five years of medical school, however, seemed out of the question. As an alternative, I briefly considered going into chemistry, but Professor Wilson argued that China was not in a condition to support people in careers in pure science at that time and recommended that I continue with medicine so as to assure myself of a reliable means of earning a livelihood. He arranged for the continuation of my Chochrane Fellowship for four more years. That meant that I had had to come up with only yuan 100 (¥100) for tuition during my entire academic career, the equivalent of about U.S. $50 at the time.

I have described these experiences in detail not because I am anyone special, but because they illustrate the enormity of the academic, financial, and linguistic obstacles faced by many young Chinese at that time in pursuing higher education. This was particularly true when one aspired to attain the best medical education available in China.

THE PUMC AS A FORCE FOR NATIONAL RENEWAL

A few words may be said about the characteristics of the PUMC from the standpoint of its early students. In the nation's capital, the

PUMC stood as a proud symbol of the authority and legitimacy of science, the scientific method of studies and scientific medical knowledge. Contained within a walled compound were a faculty of high-ranking scientists trained in the West, residential and teaching facilities for a small, hand-picked group of Chinese students, and a teaching hospital furnished with the finest and most modern facilities and technological equipment available anywhere in the world.

The elitist character of the medical college and its technological and research emphasis reflected the specific pedagogical goal of its Rockefeller Foundation sponsors. That aim was to initiate the spread of scientific medicine in a revitalized China by preparing a small vanguard of superbly trained medical educators who would provide leadership for the long-term process.

To this end, no expense had been spared in constructing or operating the teaching institution, nor were academic standards any less rigorous than at the finest scientific institutions in the West. In a later era, the college would come to be regarded as something of a showplace because no developing country could duplicate such an institution. Still, it served an undeniably important role at that time, in that the quality of its diagnostic capabilities and treatment approaches provided a model that other medical schools attempted to emulate.

EMPHASIS ON SCIENTIFIC EXCELLENCE

In eight years of intensive study at the PUMC, students gained a solid appreciation of scientific methodology and were encouraged to engage in specialized research at advanced levels. The size of the graduating classes was small: three in 1924, five in 1925, three in 1926, ten in 1927, fourteen in 1928, sixteen in 1929, and eight in 1930. Later classes were larger, although rarely exceeding twenty-five.

Limiting enrollment was deemed necessary and appropriate, despite China's then critical shortage of modern physicians, given the institutional goal of producing an elite vanguard of medical educators and administrators. Quality, not quantity, was the object. Later developments may have vindicated this judgment, although in retrospect it seems likely that a somewhat larger number of graduates could have been turned out without lowering the standard—perhaps double the number who actually completed training.

Faculty and students performed research work of high caliber. The most widely publicized of these achievements was one that produced a major archeological breakthrough: the finding, outside Beijing, of skeletal remains of an extinct species, Peking man. In another example, the development of ephedrine from *ma huang*, a plant long familiar in Chinese pharmacology, facilitated treatment of respiratory diseases the world over.[8]

Excellence was sought in the classroom as well as the laboratory. One of the best teachers I encountered, returned student and physiologist Dr. Robert S. K. Lim, earned the respect of students and colleagues alike for his facility in lecturing and laboratory experimentation. Another respected member of the faculty was Dr. Harther L. Keim, who interested me in dermatology so greatly that initially I chose this as my field of specialization.

For the development of the ideas and ideals that were to have a crucial impact on my subsequent life and accomplishments, however, it was John Grant to whom I was most in debt. He not only steered me into public health as a career but also recommended me for the position in rural health at Dingxian, where I was subsequently able to do pioneering experimentation in rural health care delivery under the aegis of the Mass Education Movement (MEM).

I regard that component of my life's work as particularly important, because it was the basis for the Dingxian model of community medicine, an innovative, new approach to the provision of rural health care marked by a fundamental reliance on village-based health practitioners. Postrevolutionary authorities were able to adapt ideas developed at Dingxian to great advantage in building a nationwide rural health care system after 1958, one that employed village-based "barefoot doctors" as its basic care providers.

The legacy of Dingxian suggests that, while the PUMC was undeniably elitist in conception, isolated within its own confines from the reality of China, some of its students nonetheless were thinking and acting along lines that went well beyond the conventional concepts of the college. A small but highly visible group of graduates, concerned about the welfare of the common people, showed no lack of imagination and initiative in using their education for the benefit of their own society.

JOHN B. GRANT: FOCUSING ON THE REALITY

John B. Grant, whom I first met as a student in 1926, later became an internationally known public health leader. As a young man he already displayed the vision, originality of thought, and tough-minded pragmatism that marked his long career.

Assigned to explore the incidence of hookworm in China as a possible starting point for Rockefeller Foundation work in our country, he concluded that developing a program limited to curative measures alone would be relatively useless in the long term. What was needed was a two-pronged program combining curative and preventive measures. Grant believed, however, that it was impossible to undertake such a program without a functioning public health organization and sufficient numbers of trained personnel, of which China had neither.[9] The critical scarcity of modern physicians in our country as disclosed in the course of Grant's investigation was one of a combination of circumstances contributing to the decision to establish the PUMC, and it followed quite naturally that he was invited, in 1921, to establish its department of public health.

Realizing that local communities had to have their own permanent health agencies if health improvement was to be sustained, Grant applied himself particularly to developing pioneer public health leadership. He encouraged interest in public health careers in as many students as possible and never lost sight of those he considered the best and the brightest. Because he had the support of the Rockefeller Foundation and the PUMC, he was able to make opportunities for those in whom he took a special interest to pursue graduate studies abroad, and once they had finished their training, he often found key positions for them in the municipal health administrations being developed with his help.

A major component of his teaching philosophy was his insistence on experience outside the classroom. As an initial step, he established a course requirement that each student organize and conduct a complete health survey in a locality of that student's own choosing. More importantly, after several years in China, Grant sought the cooperation of Beijing municipal police authorities and established an urban health station, where PUMC medical and nursing students were provided with an opportunity to practice what they learned in the classroom. The experimental Peking First

Health Station served an urban precinct of about 50,000 persons. Internship at the health station gave valuable experience to many students who later served in staff positions in China's fledgling municipal, provincial, and national health administrations.

Throughout his years in China, Grant continued to hammer at the theme of integrating preventive and curative services, couching his ideas in such a way as to point toward the concept of state, that is, nationalized medicine. The progress of health care under missionary sponsorship dissatisfied him precisely because it failed to progress far beyond the provision of hospitals and clinics and the treatment of individual patients. He wanted to see instead the rapid institution of a health care approach encompassing both preventive and curative components, and one that was adaptable to China's particular needs.

He assembled these ideas more than fifty years ago into a set of principles and practice he termed "community health care," the forerunner of present-day community medicine. According to his definition, community health care entailed "the provision of preventive and curative services, using modern epidemiological techniques in assessing the health needs of population groups, the setting of priorities, and the assessment of results achieved." Such an undertaking necessitated careful experimentation with new methods of health care and the evaluation of results, as well as the provision of a realistic setting for instruction of medical, nursing, and health science students.

In 1934, after nearly fifteen years as head of the public health department, Grant left the PUMC to assume broader responsibilities for Rockefeller-funded programs in China. His influence continued well after his departure. Between 1924 and 1942, at least 17 percent of all medical and nursing students entered the field of public health.

Grant left a pervasive and enduring mark on public health in China, reflecting an intuitive understanding of the complexity of modern society and the fundamental responsibility of medicine in its well-being. He believed that no one was better suited to solve China's grievous problems than the Chinese themselves, and that the only appropriate solutions were those within the economic reach of the community involved, not those that required outside support.

If his judgment failed him at any point, it was perhaps in under-emphasizing the value of clinical training. Most academics agreed on the paramount importance of such training, especially for a public health educator. It was difficult for anyone with inadequate clinical training to enlist public confidence or to command respect from his colleagues. Yet for reasons known only to him, Grant made arrangements for one medical student to graduate before he had served an internship of any length at all, and for another student to leave after an internship of only six months.

Looking back at my personal relationship with Grant, I see him as having been both teacher and lifelong friend. Our association not only spanned my student years at the PUMC but also several decades thereafter at a time when his professional responsibilities took him to other parts of the world.

Throughout that period, he intervened at many points to assist me in finding an appropriate position from which to experiment with new ideas about rural health development. Immediately after graduation, he drew my attention to a popular education program, where I went to work among the Chinese peasants for the first time. Later he made it possible for me to do graduate work in public health abroad. Then, after my return to China, he recommended to James Y. C. Yen, director of the Mass Education Movement, that I be offered the position of its medical director. In that post, I had the unique opportunity to do experimental work in rural health, leading to the unprecedented Dingxian health care delivery system. Many of the best years of my life were spent in close association with Grant's ideas and ideals.

STUDENTS AND THE NATIONAL AWAKENING

With their country in the midst of the National Awakening during the early 1920s, medical students in China were inevitably caught up in the ferment of the times. Along with intellectuals and workers, they provided the main impetus for protest against their own government and Japan in 1919, following the revelation that representatives at the Paris Peace Conference had accepted Japan's claim to former German holdings in Shandong Province.[10] Stung by this concession—seen as an ultimate humiliation at foreign hands, ur-

ban leaders throughout the country commenced a critical assessment of Chinese life and culture. This culminated into pressure for
the radical remaking of China along Western lines. In that call for
renewal, students played a major role.

It would have been impossible, as a student in Beijing at that
time, to have remained entirely oblivious to ongoing political and
intellectual developments. Until the spring of 1925, nonetheless,
many, if not most, PUMC students, including myself, were almost
entirely absorbed in our studies. The killing of a number of street
demonstrators by British police in Shanghai on May 30 of that year,
however, shattered our concentration, and after joining the nationwide student protests that followed, a number of us became rapidly politicized and committed to working for change.

The May 30 incident in Shanghai seems to have been a turning
point in my own life. Energies that had heretofore been applied to
academic interests were now channeled into opposition activities. I
volunteered as a teacher of politics in the middle schools and spent
time in ideological debate and discussion with new friends. Then,
as I began public health studies in the fall of 1926, heard Grant's
lectures, worked in the Beijing First Health Station, and conducted
the survey on health conditions in a rural areas, my thoughts began to crystallize. Unconsciously, I had been searching for a means
for applying the knowledge I was acquiring in medical school to
society, and the means was becoming increasingly apparent.

POLITICAL ACTIVISM AT THE PUMC

The deaths in Shanghai had fanned patriotic sentiment—already
high—to a feverish pitch, spawning a wave of strikes, protests, and
demonstrations that quickly spread to other cities. Very shortly the
Beijing Student Union called for a general strike of university and
college students to protest British imperialism and the ineptitude,
corruption, and disunity of warlord rule.

Unlike students at Beijing, Qinghua, and other universities,
PUMC undergraduates were generally quite apolitical, and until
then had never engaged in any kind of collective political action
whatsoever. Those who had attended missionary schools were, as
a group, particularly unconcerned about politics, so much so that
many seldom, if ever, read the Chinese newspapers. Nonetheless,

in this instance, a significant portion of the student body, influenced by an experience in a government school, or by a teacher, parent, relative, or friend, favored participation, even at the sacrifice of their studies.

This response caught PUMC authorities unprepared and placed them in a very difficult position. Some faculty members, while unsympathetic with the movement in any way, felt that the extent of government corruption justified the strike, and students should be allowed to participate. Certainly on balance, however, the administration would have preferred that they remain out of the fray, concentrating on academic pursuits. Dr. Heng Liu, medical administrator of the hospital and the first Chinese to hold a PUMC staff appointment, advised students not to participate.

In the end, however, the authorities capitulated, probably having no real option in the matter. They suspended classes for a few weeks and postponed the scheduled examinations. Professor Robert S. K. Lim led the PUMC contingent in the demonstrations.

As it turned out, general interest at the PUMC was rather short lived, and political activism as a whole waned rather quickly. Only a few undergraduates, myself included, continued to involve themselves in the reform effort. Factionalism and dissension within the Beijing Student Union helped to damp my enthusiasm. My own sustained interest was attributable in part to the number of stimulating intellectuals I had come to know and who offered challenging opportunities for analysis and debate. They included Dr. Xu Shilian, a professor of sociology at Yanjing University, and Chen Yuren (Eugene Chen), editor of a prominent English-language newspaper, the *People's Livelihood*, and a close political ally of Sun Yat-sen.

Preoccupied with reform issues, I failed to concentrate on preparing for final examinations in 1926 and received a poor grade in physiology. Alarmed, I once again devoted my attention exclusively to scholastic work. Lim arranged for me to make up my poor grade by assisting on a special department project. This was an exhilarating prospect. Dr. Hou Xiangchuan was delegated to train me in research, and later I had the thrill of having the work I had done under him appear in *The Chinese Journal of Physiology*, a prestigious professional publication.

By the time I completed my first year in medical school, I had already been exposed to two sides of student life, the academic and the political. As I began public health instruction under Grant in 1926, I had mixed feelings about their relative importance. On one hand, the student movement made me feel that one could not be purely technical; on the other hand, it was clear that one had always to give the lion's share of one's time and energy to academic subjects.

Relations between foreigners and Chinese were particularly fragile at that time, and students were very sensitive about the country's weakness and vulnerability. Grant taught his course in a very tactful way, however, using material he had collected in China to suggest that some of that vulnerability could be attenuated by improved socioeconomic well-being among the peasantry.

That idea was furthered by the several weeks I spent in the small village of Tongxian, a rural settlement about fifteen miles from Beijing that I had chosen to study in fulfillment of the public health requirement for a survey of rural conditions. My stay was brief. I was able to make only superficial observations of the needs of the local people and had no opportunity to experience rural life in any real sense. Still even in that brief time I saw many problems that could be improved through public health measures, while the lack of medical care and the very backward conditions in the villages left a deep impression. Other classmates had the same reaction. They began to feel that the misery of the peasants must be relieved, and that it was up to them to see that this was done.

Science and Social Conscience

Medical students in our country at that time were much attuned to the philosophical implications of the scientific knowledge they were acquiring. Sensitive students everywhere have reflected on the potential of science for the creation of a more equitable society and for the better management of human problems, and we were no exception. If anything, that special time in China's history made the question all the more important. Nevertheless, many students believed that because China's problems were so enormous, little could be done to them.

Consequently, the great majority of PUMC graduates planned

their careers without much consideration of the immense medical needs of the country at that time. Some went into teaching and others into health administration. Most, however, like other recent modern medical graduates in China at that time, settled into urban medical careers in Beijing, Shanghai, or Nanjing. The prevailing attitude in the professional community concerning the enormous public health problems in rural China was one of apathy and inertia.

Choosing a public health career, as a minority decided to do, required a strong sense of social responsibility and considerable determination. For without a patriotic and idealistic motivation, opting for such a specialization made little or no sense. The work demanded sacrifice of the academic and financial rewards of research or private practice and had to be performed under very difficult conditions. One could not settle in the relative comfort of the city. The most urgent problems—isolation, poverty, ignorance, and disease—were found in rural areas.

Forming the Binying Society

The benefits of knowledge uncovered in the age of science in the West had barely touched China's rural areas, where 80 percent of the population lived under conditions little different from those of Europe several centuries earlier. Among the peasants, nutrition was inadequate and sanitation was ignored. Conditions among the urban poor were only marginally better, if that. The seeming fixity of suffering and disease and the magnitude of need in rural areas defied attempts at solution.

At the PUMC, however, a sentiment took shape among a nucleus of idealistic students that it was not only feasible, but imperative, to try to improve the living conditions of the general population. On the basis of the existing social and political situation, there seemed to be no time to waste. Thus a small group of first-year medical students, including myself, gathered together one evening in 1926 to consider what action we could take even before we had completed our medical studies.

We organized ourselves on a formal basis as the Binying Society, choosing that name because, in the sixty-year cycle of the Chinese calendar, 1926 was the Binying year, the year of the tiger. Zhu

Changgeng was instrumental in our organizing effort. Other members included Yang Jishi, Jia Kui, and Zhu Futang, all of whom later became professors of medicine.

Defining Our Aims

Meanwhile, John Grant had introduced me to Yuan Dengli, a professor of physical education at the Normal University of Beijing. An instant rapport developed between this thoughtful older man and myself. We both knew that the backwardness of the government was an impediment to any effort to improve national health. Nonetheless, suggested Yuan, an inroad might be made through health education. If I were interested in community medicine, he said, I should think more about how this could be done. "Take, for example, typhus fever, which is raging in Beijing," he remarked. "This disease can be completely prevented by personal hygiene, provided people are aware of the danger of louse bites. Take trachoma, for another example. If one could practice personal hygiene, if people knew how to protect their eyes from infection, then this disease would be controllable." Yuan believed that such things would not require much government support and thus were practical for China at that time.

Thinking along these lines, Binying Society members rather quickly agreed that our fundamental mission would be educational. Given the focus on technical excellence at the PUMC, we might easily have been blinded by technology and its immense, and seemingly immediate, potential for relieving our country's health and medical problems. Technological development had its place in any modern order, and because the West had assigned priority to the development of technical skills and the pursuit of advanced scientific research, we might readily have chosen to follow its example.

Conditions in China, however, were very different from those in the West. Far from being fundamentally healthy, our population was disease-ridden, and life expectancy was short. Far from being clean and sanitary, our environment was rife with health hazards, to whose dangers most people were wholly oblivious. The level of health consciousness was deplorable, and every year hundreds of thousands of persons died from preventable illness.

A few medical students alone could not change that situation. Before modern medicine could be introduced and successfully implemented in such a society, people had to be provided with a fundamental appreciation of science and a scientific point of view. The prospective benefits in health improvement inherent in scientific medicine had to be made clear. Only then would it be possible to impose public pressure on the government for improved conditions.

As it was, popular beliefs and practices about illness and disease had almost medieval overtones. In rural China, because the concept of infection was almost universally unknown, cleanliness and sanitation were assigned no importance, and the spread of disease through contagion was never considered. Traditional midwives often used mud to arrest umbilical-cord bleeding. People drank unboiled water from wells just a few feet from unprotected latrines. Children with diphtheria and scarlet fever shared beds with the healthy children in the same family.

In urban China, the education and health consciousness levels were somewhat higher, but even there there was much ground to be covered. For example, missionaries, and now the government, were building and operating hospitals, but to most Chinese, including city dwellers, a hospital still was a very foreign and unfamiliar idea, and the ordinary person had no notion of how one should function, what standards should be maintained, or what was required in the way of equipment. The lack of health consciousness among the Chinese at that time may astound present-day readers, but that is, indeed, precisely what China was like at that time.

Under these circumstances, health education was clearly a critical priority. Through our public information efforts, we wanted to try to make people more knowledgeable concerning health and disease, increase their sense of personal responsibility in regard to their own health, and eliminate prevailing misconceptions about modern medicine and what it could or could not accomplish. As it was, to the extent that people thought about the difference between modern and traditional medicine at all, because most early medical missionaries had been surgeons, they tended to think that Western medicine was preferable for surgery, while traditional medicine was superior in its use of drugs.

We believed that if the public could be made aware of the fundamental differences between the two medicines and of the crucial importance of these differences, we could more quickly develop popular confidence in the new system imparted from the West. Essentially we hoped to convey the idea that scientific medicine was intrinsically set apart from our indigenous system in that it relied on the scientific method, and that scientific inquiry into the derivation of disease produced an inherent interest in prevention as a corollary to interest in treatment. Traditional medicine, by contrast, was largely indifferent to the issue of prevention.

As matters stood, aside from a few intellectuals, few Chinese at that time had any understanding of these crucial differences at all. Most people regarded modern medicine simply as something involving the prescription of medication or performance of surgery. Medical practitioners themselves contributed to this notion, perpetrating the idea that all one had to do was hang up a shingle and prescribe from a catalog of drugs or learn a few surgical techniques. If a patient recovered, the physician or the drugs that were prescribed were credited with the recovery. Seldom, if ever, did it occur to them that nursing care, rest, cleanliness, or diet might affect the outcome, much less that any patients get well by themselves without benefit of any medical input whatsoever.

Facing the Challenge

The Binying Society decided rather quickly on a plan to develop a publication to increase public awareness of health issues. We would try to persuade a leading newspaper publisher to agree to the insertion of a health supplement into copies of his newspaper on a weekly basis. It would be called *The Binying Weekly*, and I was elected its editor.

Both the missionaries and the Peking First Health Station were already undertaking some health education work. The station was training midwives and offering health education classes for schoolteachers. Its general thrust emphasized personal hygiene and maternal and child care and other topics of immediate and local interest. Its method was based on trying to involve the students directly in the learning process. We supported these ideas and believed in the program as far as it went. Our goal, however, was to try to reach a larger and more influential audience and to present some fundamental ideas about scientific medicine, rather than to teach specific techniques.

The missionaries had organized a Council on Health Education, whose plans included the education of teachers, the conducting of surveys on health conditions, and the organization of health propaganda campaigns in the streets. The hope was, whenever possible, to integrate these health education efforts with evangelistic programs. One of the best known missionary activists in health education was W. W. Peter.

Of the various missionary health education efforts, the most visible were their street campaigns, which were based on a strategy of arousing curiosity through audiovisual aides, mechanical devices, and occasionally, parades using floats and megaphones. This could be accomplished with some effect in cities and towns, but in outlying areas, there was no electricity with which to operate equipment. In any event when the campaigns were over, they were soon forgotten.

Accordingly, the idea of a newspaper supplement appealed to us on two counts. It would be a sustained, rather than sporadic effort, and it would appeal to a sizable and influential group of readers, rather than a disparate group of bystanders in the street.

In laying our plans, we were thinking specifically of trying to reach other medical students and graduate physicians. We were greatly disturbed by the prevailing inertia in the medical profession concerning our country's grave health problems, and we wanted to make our citizenry more aware that the national interest in health was their own. As it was, the concept of public responsibility was quite alien to those physicians who had not been exposed to the classical tradition. This was particularly unfortunate in view of the backwardness of the common people, who were poor and needy and who could be taken advantage of rather easily.

Our planning for the publication was also premised on the recognition that a group of medical students alone could not possibly bring about significant improvement in health conditions. Our chief hope lay in being able to arouse influential intellectuals to take a stand on various health issues and bring pressure on the officials. We thus hoped to stimulate interest among readers whose views carried weight with the warlord regime as well as the general public.

Differences among members of the Binying Society had arisen initially as to what topics we should address. Some members favored very specific topical material, others a more generalized approach. Soon, however, we agreed that our first job was to help people understand what modern medicine was all about. We would be wasting our time talking about specifics, we concluded, before people understood some basic ideas. As it was, the Chinese public as a whole had not yet been introduced to such ideas as that that disease is transmittable; that infection occurs when microbes enter the body, gain a foothold, and multiply; and that wounds thus must be kept clean. Until we provided some basic groundwork in scientific principles, there was no use in teaching basic health practices, because anything that was not understood and appreciated would hardly be followed.

Moreover, if we taught people such things without first establishing the cause-and-effect relationships involved, they might not carry out our instructions properly, and in some cases the consequences could be dangerous. Once a basic education in scientific principles had been conveyed, we could teach the techniques rather rapidly.

The idea of a weekly newspaper supplement on health was quite innovative, but because it was without precedent, no newspaper publisher was easily convinced of its feasibility, much less its ultimate value. Obtaining publisher cooperation was difficult also because neither their editorial boards nor their readers regarded health topics as being of much importance. Worse still, there was a large market for patent medicine, prepared and sold by persons with little or no medical training, and newspaper editors were quite naturally more interested in the income derived from advertisements of these products than in subsidizing our efforts.

Much to our delight, though, we succeeded in time in getting the widely circulated and rather important *Peking World Herald* to agree to include our supplement. The paper already had several other supplements on different subjects. To obtain the publisher's agreement, we had to furnish all the material, for he had originally refused to consider our idea, saying that he had no one to write it. There was another problem, too. We had hoped to ask various prominent physicians and others to contribute articles. However, scientifically trained physicians proved to be unwilling, in many

cases, to submit articles for editorial review by persons who themselves lacked any background in science. Even those who were
willing, being unaccustomed to writing for a popular audience,
often were unable to make themselves understood. So we ended
up soliciting material from other medical students but by and large
writing most of the articles ourselves. This required a sacrifice of
time, energy, and other interests. It became very difficult to sustain
our efforts while trying to keep up with our medical studies. The
drain on our energies was tremendous, and we found ourselves
working day and night to keep the publication going.

The *Peking World Daily* published the supplement until 1927,
when political affairs preempted its news space, and the medical
supplement was discontinued. *New China*, a scientific journal,
picked up the idea, and we hoped to continue to collaborate with it
on a permanent basis. Just two months after this arrangement began, however, its editors decided to suspend publication of all
supplements. We then moved to *Da Gong Bao*.

In time, the supplement gained recognition. It appeared regularly for five years, proffering hundreds of informative articles. A
number of PUMC students contributed material, and some faculty
members gave us encouragement. Of course, others thought that
we were wasting our time. Even among students who wished us
well, however, support was only nominal at best. A few students
disapproved outright, regarding our activities as appropriate to a
politician, but not to a scientist. Disappointment at this attitude
was offset by success. When we began to receive letters from a
number of intellectuals, we were convinced that our impact was
growing. As the audience for the supplement increased, some articles prompted popular demands on the government for improvement in health services.

Content

Just a few excerpts from the supplement are presented here; readers who desire more may consult the files in the national library.
Some of the views expressed are dated, and some of the problems
that we raised have been resolved or become less important. Still,
the material is of some importance; if for no other reason, it suggests what a small group of students at a leading medical college

in China were thinking five decades ago and how many of the problems they wrote about are relevant in developing countries today.

One concern of the editors was to rid modern, scientific medicine of the disadvantage of being regarded as "foreign." At that time, it was common in our country, and still is today to some extent, to distinguish between so-called Western medicine and Chinese medicine. This tendency is unfortunate as it obscures the true, temporal basis for distinguishing between the two systems, one associated with ancient learning and the other with modern knowledge. While refraining from judgments about which system was superior, we wanted the public to think, not in terms of Chinese as contrasted with Western medicine, but in terms of ancient as contrasted with modern medicine.

> Medicine and medical knowledge belong to the whole world. Our people, deeply committed to traditional medicine, call the newly-introduced medicine from the West "western" medicine. This is natural, but actually in the West, there is only the difference between ancient and modern medicine.[11]

What was at issue, we tried to suggest, was not a value judgment between things Eastern and Western. That is, we were not arguing for "respecting medicine from abroad and despising our own." Rather, it was a case of wanting our population to benefit from the application of scientific medical knowledge, as Japan had done. "Japan . . . has adopted modern medicine to the best advantage of its own people. This does not mean [however] that modern medicine has reached a stage of perfection."[12] For that matter, we felt that there were shortcomings in either system. We believed it was foolish to assume that favorable outcomes resulted from modern medical treatment simply because there was some scientific justification for its application. We tried to emphasize to people that in modern or traditional medicine there is always an element in the outcome that is attributable to pure chance.

> It is therefore important to tell the common people that chance sometimes plays an important role in determining their (confidence) in either one system or the other. We do not mean by that that traditional medicine cures disease by chance, and modern medicine all by scientific knowledge.[13]

We wanted to discourage blind faith in either one system or the other.

In the midst of the growing controversy between the two medicines, *The Binying Weekly* argued for equitable treatment. We editorialized that if regulations applied to one type of practice, they should apply to the other: "The Society is not sympathetic with the government in enforcing the kind of laws and regulations governing only the practice of traditional medicine."[14] We suggested that it was impractical to propose to deny traditional practioners the right to practice because "their number is quite large, and there are no available substitutes."[15] We asserted that there was value in both systems and proposed "the establishment of an institute of research on Chinese drugs, and also an academy of traditional medicine."[16]

Opponents of traditional medicine at that time were charging that some of its practitioners were incompetent. As its editor, I pointed out that this could be said of modern medicine as well:

> Now if we examine the status of so-called practitioners of modern medicine we may discover that they are quite varied in quality. One is composed of graduates of regular medical schools, of which only a few are well-equipped and staffed with well-trained people. Another group is composed of apprentices of missionary doctors; a third is composed of charlatans practicing so-called western medicine. As long as the last two groups are still practicing in the community, they bring disrepute to modern medicine. Medical control with uniform criteria for all practitioners is essential.

> Our government should organize formal health education in normal, primary, and secondary schools, and also should promulgate laws governing not only medical practitioners, but also the use of drugs.

> The government, in formulating laws, must proceed gradually, however. Without informed public opinion, laws are bound to meet with resistance. At the same time, we should also know that many schools of modern medicine must be strengthened. Our government should emphasize careful planning in education and law.[17]

Editorial attention focused on many other topics besides the encounter between two medicines. Because hospitals were regarded as nothing more than places where medications were dispensed or surgery performed, other matters that directly affected the patient such as diet, nursing care, and sanitary standards received little or no attention. The teaching hospital of the PUMC was excellent, of course, reputed to be the best equipped and best managed hospital in East Asia. Other hospitals were not so good, however. The editor described conditions a visitor to a Beijing hospital encountered in 1927:

> When I raised the curtain of the entrance, I saw my friend, Mr. Shen, and a man—not a nurse—was handing him two bowls of rice. My friend looked pale and weak, and was breathing rapidly. In that room, there were two beds; one had a mosquito net and the other did not. There were a few packages of drugs on the table and a bottle of fluid without instructions. Each package had a label which read "one package three times daily." While I talked to my friend, a few flies buzzed around in the room. I learned that the bedding was brought in by the patients without delousing. I used my hand to feel my friend's body and found that his chest and abdomen were covered with sweat, showing me he had never had a bath in the hospital.[18]

Since the government and the public at that time were aware of the need for hospitals, they were willing to fund them. Yet given the public tolerance for such conditions, the expenditures were almost self-defeating.

Another topic in which the editor was particularly interested was rural health care. A 1929 article pointed out that preventable illness was responsible in great part for the high mortality rates:

> If our health conditions could be improved to the degree comparable to those of many countries, we could probably cut the number of deaths by one half. The unnecessary loss of people is grievous to our economy and is a sign of a backward civilization.

> Since 80 or more percent of those who die each year unnecessarily occur among the farming people, we naturally should pay close attention to [that group]. [At one time I] thought there were not many patients in the villages. After working in two rural communities, however I began to realize there were actually many sick persons in the countryside.

> [When rural people became ill] they usually pray before gods, and if minor ailments get better, they say the gods cured the disease. Patients with serious ailments usually get worse due to delayed treatment. They first try herbs and patent medicine. They rarely use, and cannot afford to use, formal or so-called official medicine, which is drugs prescribed by scholar-doctors. Some patients we see at [modern medical] clinics mostly have tried witchcraft, conventional herbs, patent medicine, and traditional medicine without success.

The peasants generally believe that sickness is due to bad luck or lack of adaptation to water and soil [the ecological conditions]. They do not know that each disease has its own cause. Traditional medicine generally does not know the real cause of disease, and nothing can be said about prevention. . . . Smallpox, which had disappeared in some countries, is still prevalent in our villages. Diseases like smallpox and cholera are quite easily preventable; there is urgent need for a rural health service practicing scientific medicine.[19]

We noted, too, that the disinterest of modern physicians in rural practice contributed to the problem:

Graduates of modern medical schools do not go to poor villages to make a living. Government appointed doctors are unwilling to work in rural areas. Therefore, the peasant when sick, cannot get regular treatment. Patients travel two or three miles to see a doctor in a rural clinic. This shows the extreme shortage of doctors and medicine in our countryside.

Although we have thousands of doctors in the cities, in the villages of North China 40 percent of our people have no medical facilities of any kind. Western medicine has been in China for almost a century and only cities have slight contact with it.[20]

Another issue that interested the society was government responsibility for public health, and in that context we stressed the importance of effective health administration. We felt that even at that time health care should not be left entirely in the hands of private practitioners, and that it was time to introduce state-supported medicine.

An effective public health administration, of course, required appropriately trained professional personnel, of which there was a great scarcity. We might begin to remedy this glaring weakness, the editor felt, by using normal schools as a channel of health education for the general public. An actual health officer, in *The Binying Weekly*, recommended that such a practitioner "should be a graduate of a good medical school; have special training in public health with understanding of local health conditions; have good character; and be capable, with leadership qualities." The health officer further stated:

Lack of health knowledge is a [common problem] and a great obstacle to the operation of the Public Health Administration. The Beijing Municipality has both high and ordinary normal schools, which are the best places for systematic health education. An important duty of the health officer is to train teachers and those preparing to be teachers. When young students have been trained by competent teachers with the proper teaching material, they will be educated from the standpoint of personal health and public health. Only then can the Public Health Administration advance satisfactorily.[21]

Editorial attention was also given to persuading readers that public health is a national asset:

Statistic[al] evidence shows clearly the relationship between health and productivity. People do not appreciate the economic value of health, but health can be shown as a great economic asset for a nation whose level of productivity is pitifully low.

It is easy to understand the economic value of a working individual in relation to his family, but it is hard to visualize the economic value of community health to the entire nation. . . . In our country, the number of deaths due to preventable disease is estimated to be as high as 6 million per year. Cases of illness that could have been prevented accounted for almost 2 million. The economic loss calculated even at the present level of productivity must be enormous.

If infectious diseases such as typhoid fever, tuberculosis, diphtheria, and tetanus could be prevented, many lives would be saved, and socio-economic loss would be greatly reduced. . . . So if our government and our people appreciate the objectives and techniques of preventive medicine, and practice them through organized community efforts, it would contribute to the prosperity of our country. The economic value of health is enormous, and requires much study to elucidate its significance.[22]

Finally, but perhaps most important of all, the *Binying Weekly* stressed the requirement for a spirit of social responsibility and of personal sacrifice among members of the medical profession. In one article the editor noted that he, too, like everyone else, had lacked the appropriate attitude when entering the field:

When I began to study medicine, I considered the duty of the medical profession to be "hanging up shingles" and prescribing drugs for patients.

[But] at 25, I have come to believe that medicine is not a profession over and above society. It is only a part of social enterprise. This seems to be a change of personal attitude on my part. For myself, without this change, I never would have decided to shift my direction of clinical medicine to social medicine and village life; and I would not discuss rural health with my readers.

For the last two years, I have believed that health without education cannot be practiced effectively and education without health is in vain.[23]

The Binying Society felt the need not only to popularize medical knowledge but also to

> help medical schools draw closer to society . . . through this weekly, the medical profession is expected to develop the real spirit of modern medicine, which includes correct diagnosis, treatment, and extension of preventive measures. It should also try to extend the use of various diagnostic techniques. . . . Medical students should cultivate a spirit of sacrifice so as to protect the people's health. The government must take responsibility to support them especially since public health personnel should be employed in government institutions. . . . We as students of medicine have to broaden our vision and do our best to advocate the justified claim of the people for protection of their health.[24]

In another article, we noted:

> In recent years, our country has suffered from internal and external troubles and people of all walks of life could not do their business peacefully. Our country is in danger. In the field of medicine, many returned students from Germany and America are in private practice. Some young doctors consider private practice as only a means to serve rich people and yet they still think they are not depending upon others to make a living. They are not trying to adapt what they have learned from abroad to our own conditions, showing that they do not truly appreciate the spirit of modern medicine. In particular they do not feel the responsibility for educating the younger generation in the proper way.[25]

From the standpoint of progressive thinking, the work of the society is of historic interest. Its record attests to what a few inspired young persons could accomplish at a time when the medical community as a whole was marked by inertia. That may be why, twenty five years later, Ho Chen, Vice-Minister of Health in the newly established People's Republic of China, commented to me in his office during the first national conference on health: "We know of your work in the past and look forward to your cooperation."

Nonetheless, a few decades later the Binying Society and its work seemed to have faded into oblivion. Personal collections of the supplement were largely destroyed during the Cultural Revolution. Only one complete set remained in the National Library at

Beijing. Many of the original members were deceased, and few traces remained to alert scholars writing about the PUMC to the dedicated effort a few students had engaged in voluntarily, at considerable sacrifice of time and energy, to educate the public in health matters.

How much the Binying Society and its publications contributed to the reputation of the PUMC, therefore, is an open question. At a minimum, however, its existence may have helped later generations to see that the school was far more than a mere philanthropic institution populated by a community of scholars interested only in technical excellence. It offered evidence of concern with the broad concept of human welfare as well, requiring the support of the founders as well as the motivation of a few idealistic students to keep it going over quite a few years.

3

Pioneering in Rural Health Development

In the early 1930s, fresh from graduate study in the United States and Germany, I finally had an opportunity to experiment on a health system to reach the villagers. I was invited to become director of the Department of Rural Health of the Mass Education Movement (MEM), a privately sponsored experimental program aimed at improving rural life in China by nurturing self-reliance among the peasants through popular education and other reform measures.

The MEM operated in various parts of the country. Its headquarters, however, were in Dingxian, a rural district and town of the same name, less than 100 miles from Beijing. I worked at Dingxian from 1932 to 1938, developing the health program of the movement in close association with its founder, James Y. C. Yen.

With respect to medical relief and health protection, rural China presented a bleak picture. Communicable disease was widespread, death rates were high, and life expectancy was short. Hospital- and clinic-centered missionary medicine had had little impact. Traditional practitioners, relying mainly on herbs, provided essentially the only available form of medical relief. A sense of the importance of cleanliness and sanitation was conspicuously absent, even among the few rural inhabitants who had some sort of education.

The MEM had begun simply as a popular education program, but it soon became evident that increasing literacy alone would do little to raise the standard of living. Accordingly, the program expanded as it matured, developing an integrated, multifaceted approach to rural reconstruction based on correlated programs for social change in related areas of village life. From education it moved quite naturally into agriculture and from there into health. As it undertook an increasing number of measures essentially in the public domain, the MEM tried to strengthen its relationship to central and district authorities so as to build up their cooperation and to develop a sense of government responsibility in these areas.

My particular task was to devise, through experimentation, a model system affording health protection and modern medical relief to rural Chinese, suitable for adoption in any one of the country's numerous and diverse rural districts. Nothing of the sort had been contemplated, much less tried, before. Not only was there no previous experience to guide us but also the paucity of resources in the rural areas, both economic and technical, taxed our inventiveness to the hilt.

Notwithstanding the difficulties, hard work and sacrifice were rewarded with success. By 1934, little over two years after beginning our work, we had developed a systematic rural health care organization so well regarded that the new central government in Nanjing had recommended its adoption throughout the entire country. By 1937, when hostilities with Japan forced us to cease operations, we had worked out further refinements in the system and had been operating a rural field training site for medical and nursing students for several years. More than a few international health leaders had come to Dingxian to observe our work.

In devising that first systematic rural health organization, we had been careful to avoid simply copying what the missionaries had done in urban China. That, we were convinced, would have been a grave error. Missionary medicine, after all, had evolved under conditions very different from those in rural China. Its accent on private practice and hospital- and clinic-centered practice met the needs of a privileged urban elite that shared something in common with Western society but not those of the great mass of villagers.

Our system, a versatile one that could be adapted to varying social, economic, and regional conditions, differed from the missionary model in several crucial respects. It addressed the problems of an impoverished, ill-educated, and predominantly agricultural society. It focused on the concerns of not individual patients, but entire communities, making their economic limitations its first consideration. Our rural health system also provided the benefits of advanced medical knowledge not only to a tiny segment of society, but to a vast rural population, which it linked for the first time to key centers of scientific medicine in the cities.

PRELIBERATION CHINA: 1928 to 1937

While infighting among warlords had prevailed in North China, concurrently in South China, two groups had sought to unify and stabilize the country under their own authority: The Guomindang party, led until his death in 1925 by Sun Yat-sen, and the Chinese Communist party (CCP) founded in 1921 chiefly by leading scholars and activists of the May Fourth Movement.[1] Befriended by the Soviet Union, the Guomindang and the CCP had formed a revolutionary alliance that from a base in Guangzhou for a time had imposed a modicum of unity in South China.

Like many other young people at that time, we medical students in Beijing were fed up with the constant struggle among the warlords and hoped for their defeat. We believed that China must be unified, and that Sun Yat-sen offered a leadership that would be concerned with the welfare of the people. Our high expectations were based on his political philosophy, which centered on "Three Principles of the People": "people's rights," "democracy," and "people's livelihood."

Regarding the tie between the Guomindang and the CCP, we knew that the latter had been organized in 1921, and that it conducted activities in many cities, including Shanghai, Wuhan, and even Beijing. We were aware, too, that the Soviet Union was supporting the CCP rather than the alliance as such; however, we had little knowledge of ideological differences between the CCP and the Guomindang. All that we were conscious of was that the two groups seemd to be working effectively together in the interest of the country, and so we supported the alliance.

Sun Yat-sen died in 1925, however, and after his military commander, Chiang Kai-shek, launched a successful expedition into central China, our attitude toward the Guomindang began to change. For the success of the drive into central and then North China enabled Chiang Kai-shek to broaden his personal power base, whereupon he turned on his former Communist allies, and with all the forces at his command. After bitter fighting, the Communists eventually withdrew from their urban enclaves, regrouping along the border of Hunan and Jiangxi Provinces, where they struggled to maintain a territorial foothold in various "revolutionary bases" or "liberated regions." In 1928 Chiang Kai-shek proclaimed his authority over the entire country and established a new central government in Nanjing.

Whatever expectations early supporters of the Guomindang party might have had that a Nationalist government would govern in accordance with the Three Principles were quickly dashed. Leaders gave only lip service to the formula on which the party had been founded, and as far as the needs of rural China were concerned, authorities in Nanjing showed little concern. The only departure from this pattern appeared after 1932, in the aftermath of a series of defeats suffered by Guomindang troops in unsuccessful attempts to wipe out the remaining pockets of CCP strength in rural areas. This seems to have produced the conclusion at the apex of power that some concessions might have to be made for the sake of stability in rural areas.

In one manifestation of this new strategy, the National Economic Council, under the direction of T. V. Soong, brought in several League of Nations experts to survey the situation in rural areas. One of them was Andrija Stampar, an internationally known public health leader, who visited us at Dingxian. Stampar apparently did apprise the group of the urgency of nutrition, sanitation, and health care needs in the villages, although what his specific recommendations might have been I do not know.

THE SHAPING OF HEALTH POLICY AND ADMINISTRATION

A new constitution called for the establishment of five *yuan*, or public bodies, including an executive yuan encompassing various ministries to carry out administrative functions.[2] From the standpoint of the medical profession, the establishment of a Ministry of Health—the first central health administration the country had ever had—was marked progress.

It soon became clear, however, that this had been a more or less perfunctory step. The portfolio of the ministry was given to a war-lord as a token of appreciation for his support of the party. Party leaders took little interest in the new agency and did not significantly participate in its activities.

In a sense, their indifference turned out to be a blessing in disguise, for the new minister looked to the PUMC and John Grant for help in formulating evolving health policy and in staffing his new agency. Grant was able to place several highly competent people in key positions. J. Heng Liu, for example, director of the PUMC hospital, was asked to serve as vice minister. Grant also guided the establishment of new municipal and province-level health administrations, placing many former students in these agencies as well.

Through Grant's activities and those of other current and former students and faculty members, the Rockefeller Foundation and the PUMC were able to exercise a substantial influence on evolving health policy and administration. Ties between the college and the world beyond the campus compound expanded considerably as compared with the era of the warlords.

During the decade from 1928 to 1937 there was a considerable amount of progress in the development of urban health care facilities and training institutions. Central, provincial, and municipal authorities opened hospitals and clinics. Missionary hospitals and other care agencies remained on the scene. Medical education facilities flourished as government and private groups opened new training centers. Much of this new urban aggregate developed randomly, however, without benefit of systematic planning in respect to real needs and conditions.

There was slight progress in rural areas. After 1934, for example, a few county hospitals were established. My own appointment to oversee health affairs for the Rural Normal School Movement in Xiaozhuang, too, resulted from the instigation of the central Ministry of Health. By and large, however, rural areas received little attention.

Graduate training in public health abroad was made available to a number of present and future health administrators through a program of government-sponsored fellowships and, at the instigation of John Grant, by the Rockefeller Foundation. Between 1929 and 1942, two dozen PUMC graduates were selected and sent to schools of public health in the United States. In 1930/31 I was able to complete a year's graduate work at the Harvard University School of Public Health and to pursue further work at Das Reichshaus für Hygienische Volksbelehrung in Dresden.

For a student like myself, coming from a country whose conditions were very unlike those in the United States, the Harvard experience had both positive and negative aspects. Various teachers—including Milton J. Rosenau, Edwin D. Wilson, and at the Massachusetts Institute of Technology, Clair E. Turner—exposed me to analytical and theoretical material that exerted an important influence on my thinking as a public health specialist. The field training was disappointing, however. It consisted mainly of superficial observation, without much student participation, a decided contrast to the highly motivating, hands-on exposure to the health problems of ordinary people we had had at the Peking First Health Station.

In any event, to return to medical affairs in China under Nationalist rule, in 1928 Robert S. K. Lim was elected president of the Chinese Medical Association (CMA). By that time there was, to all intents and purposes, only this one association of modern physicians, rather than two competing groups, and from Lim's election forward, its leadership was dominated by Chinese nationals. Lim took over the CMA at a time when missionary influence in it was fading and, under his direction, its emphasis became scientific rather than chiefly social. Within a short time span, the CMA began to have a major impact on health policy and administration. By 1935, the CMA had 1,700 members.

Two types of individuals accounted for its expansive influence on public health in the 1928–1937 period: (1) medical scientists with a broad orientation, of the type represented by Lim, a British-educated physiologist; and (2) physicians specifically trained in public health, such as Dr P. Z. Jin. As noted, Lim was elected to the presidency in 1928. Japanese-trained Jin, who held a high-ranking post in the health ministry, was elected to the presidency in 1935. Both men played prominent roles in shaping health policy and administration through activities both within and outside the CMA. The country was fortunate to have had such public health–minded leadership at that time, for without them the influential CMA would have been much more concerned with pure technology, contributing very little to the more important topics of medical education and health protection.

As it was, they infused the association with their public health–oriented outlook. A public health committee became active in prevention of tuberculosis, venereal disease, and cholera and in promotion of maternal and child health. There was some interest in rural health and issues in medical education, in which I actively participated. There were actions to press the membership to support the central Ministry of Health in implementing various health measures. The committee also developed criteria for evaluation of the evolving municipal health administrations.

The shift within the organization to a more professional emphasis was further evidenced in the scholarly upgrading of the association's publication, *The Chinese Medical Journal.* In part the more scholarly content of the journal reflected the high quality of research by students at the PUMC, who contributed quite a few articles. The PUMC staff members also exercised an influence on medical affairs at that time through the CMA and the journal.

Nurses were also becoming influential health activists. The 1930 CMA meeting was held jointly with the Chinese Nursing Association. By this time 32 nurses had completed training at the PUMC, and 200 attended the joint meeting. By now nurses were so involved with public health activity that collaboration with them was seen as an important step forward, indicating growing recognition of the profession and a trend toward upgrading quality.

All told, during this period, the impact of the activities of physicians, nurses, and academicians associated with the CMA on public health and medical affairs was very strong. This circumstance was attributable in part to the new, businesslike and scientific orientation of the professional organization and also to generalized close collaboration with the government.

Whatever doubts the CMA or other agencies working for social change at that time may have had regarding the ruling clique in the Guomindang, they were compelled to work closely with, as well as within, the bureaucracy. Otherwise they could not have accomplished much, for in that period a private organization without connections in the government counted for very little. Before 1928 such recommendations on public health as the CMA had made to government authorities had usually been ignored, whereas in the 1928–1937 period, they were more usually accepted and implemented.

A positive step in the planning area in the 1928–1937 period was the formation by representatives of the Ministry of Health and the Ministry of Education of a Joint Commission for Medical Education. Its aim was to bring about some uniformity in the highly diverse medical training programs of various private and public medical colleges. The commission eventually recommended a standardized six-year medical curriculum, including a one-year internship in all medical colleges. This appeared to be quite adequate for the country at the time.

While the trends in health policy and administration that evolved in the Nanjing decade were generally favorable to long-term national well-being—although the rural population had as yet benefited little from the process—in one respect these trends were not favorable. The adverse relationship between some members of the modern medical community and traditional scholar-physicians escalated to new heights after World War I and erupted into open controversy during the 1920s and early 1930s.

The struggle between the two systems of medicine had become quite fierce even before the Guomindang had established itself in Nanjing. As noted, a minority of returned students and missionary medical supporters, convinced that traditional medicine was worthless, had organized a systematic campaign for its abolition. In the mid-1920s they had written scathing attacks in the press and had pressed through the CMA for measures to curtail its practice or teaching.

In 1928 they found some allies in the new Nationalist health bureacracy who shared their point of view, and were willing to further it through the promulgation of official rulings. For example, the ministries of health and of education issued a joint regulation decreeing that traditional practitioners must term their patient care facilities "clinics" rather than hospitals and their training institutions "courses" rather than schools of medicine. The regulations seemed to be aimed at diminishing the credibility of traditional medicine.

The regulations aroused strong resentment from scholar-physicians who, as a group, had important political connections of their own in the government and who, because of their high social standing and press connections, were in a favorable position to mold public opinion. They immediately organized a protest meeting in Shanghai that drew a large attendance from many provinces. The conferees agreed to send a petition of protest to the Guomindang leadership and to dispatch a delegation to meet with officials of the central executive yuan in Nanjing. One of their most powerful backers was Chen Guofu, friend and confidante of Chiang Kai-shek and a powerful figure in the Guomindang.

The long-term impact of the organization of scholar-physicians in their collective interest was substantial. The most significant outcome was the organization in 1930 of a Bureau of Traditional Medicine on a level with the Ministry of Health in the central government. Another important result was impetus given to the establishment of new institutions providing formal training in traditional medicine.

STEPS TOWARD RURAL HEALTH ORGANIZATION

The emergence of central, provincial, and municipal health administrations and facilities and the expansion of hospitals, clinics, and teaching institutions during this period was an essentially urban phenomenon. In the rest of the country, to all intents and purposes, there was no public health organization. In fact, the expansion of health services in the cities only served to highlight the gap between urban and rural China, which was by far the most important of the many lines of social division prevailing in the country at that time.

Traditionally the rural population had been left more or less to fend for itself and for better or worse, it was county officialdom, rather than the provincial or central administration, that touched the lives of the millions of peasants. Above that level, the government had been too remote to concern itself with the people. Below it, it had been too weak. Even after the Republican Revolution of 1911, provincial governors continued to depend on district magistrates to maintain order and collect taxes.

The magistrates often ruled harshly, prizing obedience, and rarely showing interest in the improvement of the lives of their constituents. Peasants were left to educate themselves as best they could, and illiteracy was considered an individual problem. Peasants worked hard year after year but earned barely enough to support their families. Their fate lay in the hands of the district magistrate and the local landed gentry and as far as they were concerned, could be ameliorated only through prayers to various gods for intervention. In most of China, the lives of the peasants had a feudal quality, no less marked by poverty and disease at the time I went to work in Dingxian than in previous centuries.

There was no way of knowing what health conditions were like at that time in the few Communist-controlled areas. As far as the Communist fighting forces were concerned, the primary requirement was surgical care for the wounded. Also, it was critical to the fortunes of the CCP to prevent the outbreak of a devastating epidemic, which could bring a serious setback to the Revolution. In 1931, therefore, to assure an adequate number of medical personnel, the fighting forces organized their own medical school.

Probably these medical personnel shared what resources could be spared with the local peoples. Most party members, including Mao Zedong himself, were of rural origin and understood the problems of the peasants on the basis of their own experience. Moreover, they valued good relations with the farmers, for the rural masses, rather than urban workers, were now seen as the future source of party strength.

It is only assumed that the CCP gave some medical assistance to the peasants in South China with whom they came in contact. It is well known, however, that in the area of North China to which the Communists repaired in 1936, after the circuitous and costly Long March, they organized rural health care services in three provinces. By that time the Nanjing government had already recommended the Dingxian model as the prototype for systematic rural health organization around the country, but it is not known whether information about our innovative work was available in the party-controlled areas at that time.

XIAOZHUANG AND THE RURAL NORMAL SCHOOLS

The interlude between graduation from the PUMC in 1929 and the start of my work in Dingxian had included two professionally valuable experiences. One was the aforementioned academic year at Harvard for advanced public health studies in 1930/31. The other was an experience that preceded that, coming in 1929, immediately after graduation—my first full-time position in public health, when I served as Chief of the Xiaozhuang Rural Health Demonstration Program.

Like the MEM, the Rural Normal School Movement at Xiaozhuang was an ongoing popular education movement. Its founder, Tao Zhixing, was convinced, as was Jimmy Yen, of the need to educate the peasantry. Nothing, he thought, was more central to any attempt to improve their lives, and it was important, he believed, to integrate that education with the actual day-to-day realities of their lives. Whereas Yen focused on adult education, however, Tao believed in starting with children. Before this could be done, teachers had to be trained, so he began by organizing a network of rural normal schools with affiliated primary schools where future teachers could practice their skills.

As a medical student interested in health education, I had found myself very interested in Tao's philosophy and activities, and as editor of *The Binying Weekly* I had written a number of articles calling attention to the Rural Normal School Movement. At the time, *The Binying Weekly* was being well received. We had drawn favorable response from many readers and no doubt had succeeded to some degree in making people more knowledgeable about medicine and disease. Nevertheless, I was beginning to think we needed to reach a larger audience and that, by whatever means we found of doing so, it should emphasize experimentation, demonstration, and popular participation. People should be able to actually see the benefits modern medicine could bring, rather than just reading about them.

In that context, the Rural Normal School Movement was of great interest as a potential vehicle for the education of a large, rural population in the basics of modern medical knowledge. A quotation from a 1929 editorial suggests its promise:

This . . . movement has attracted the attention of many people, as the education there is not limited to teaching children how to read, but teaching them how to live as well.

As Tao remarked to the editor:

Health is the starting point of life. Rural education should emphasize health protection. Primary schools and kindergartens should consider health as the most important part of education. If a child cannot live long and remain healthy, what is the use of education.

Educators like Dr. Tao Zhixing," I wrote, "know well how important health is for education. If teachers in the villages do not try hard to promote health, the future of rural health would have no real foundation. . . . Rural school teachers are persons directly responsible for rural health at a time when our government is unable to develop rural health in general.[3]

Because of the respect I had for Tao, I welcomed the offer that I received after graduation in 1929 to develop a rural health demonstration program at Xiaozhuang. This was an early milestone in my career. The prevalence of conditions that could have been prevented or relieved by modern medical treatment among the children there impressed me very deeply.

Coming on the heels of my experience as a student taking the health survey in Tongxian, this rural health demonstration program reinforced my nascent sense of personal responsibility to the common people. I became increasingly concerned with the medical problems of the villagers, and I saw that I could do a great deal in the countryside with my valuable training. Possibly I could even accomplish more to improve the health of the people by remaining in a rural setting than by getting into urban health administration.

At Xiaozhuang, my approach to my work was premised on Tao's notion of integrating education with life reality and relied heavily on demonstration and participation. I provided the future teachers of primary schools with an introduction to the fundamentals of modern medicine, developing my own syllabus for the course. The emphasis was on prevention. They seemed to welcome this as an enrichment of their general educational background.

Far more engrossing to them, however, were the clinical sessions, where they observed me as I worked and often participated in what was taking place. We undertook a smallpox vaccination program that they heartily endorsed, knowing that the disease was often fatal or left survivors with ugly scars. They were amazed at my delivery of a dead fetus by means of decapitation. What may have impressed them most, however, was a rather inventive method I devised to treat and prevent the recurrence of ringworm of the scalp, a commonplace problem among the primary-school children. The teachers were astonished at the results, and the students who suffered from it were very happy. They were rid of a condition that had produced an offensive odor, prejudicing the teachers and other students against them.

Besides the many conditions in Xiaozhuang that required the attention of a trained physician, however, I soon discovered that there were many other conditions against which action could be taken even in the absence of a trained physician. Teachers or others could be instructed in first aid. Habits of cleanliness could be impressed on the villagers. Vaccinations and disinfectants could be offered. Water supplies and sanitation could be improved. Observations on these matters at Xiaozhuang may have germinated the ideas I developed subsequently at Dingxian to train village health workers to take on some of these relatively simple tasks.

Dingxian and the Mass Education Movement

Before going to Xiaozhuang, and later to the United States for advanced public health training, I had become somewhat conversant with the history and objectives of the Mass Education Movement. John Grant had brought James Y. C. Yen to the PUMC to speak one evening, when I was still an undergraduate.

From my own reading, I knew that Yen, who had been educated at Yale University in the United States, had gone to France during World War I to serve as a YMCA aide among 160,000 or so Chinese contract workers recruited to augment the civilian labor force. The recruits were largely illiterate, but industrious, and eager to learn to read and write. So Yen devised a teaching method based on the use of 1,000 selected Chinese characters. Familiarity with these few basic characters, he believed, would enable the men to understand a simple newspaper article, to write letters home, and eventually to learn something through reading that could improve the quality of their lives. He called his text *The One Thousand Characters*.

On returning to China after the war, Yen was able to expand his literacy program, notwithstanding the fragmentation of the country under various regional military leaders whose cooperation he managed to obtain. By the early 1920s, the MEM had become a recognized national movement, with branches in all major cities. Given its essentially rural ethos, however, it was more appropriate for the movement to have a base in rural areas, so Yen moved to Dingxian, not far from Beijing. His organization collected support from sympathetic intellectuals, local officials, and the landed gentry. Also he secured partial funding from the Milbank Memorial Fund in the United States and numerous personal contacts at home and abroad.

Not long into his efforts in Dingxian, Yen began to question the impact of a program aimed at making the peasants literate, while ignoring their dire poverty, ill health, and other problems. "We can feed their minds, but not their stomachs," he lamented to a friend. Education, he soon concluded, must be tackled together with other facets of social work. He then started to plan for a broader social experiment, where an integrated program of reconstruction could be developed and tested under educated leadership. The MEM expanded into other realms—agriculture, transport, and the establishment of rural cooperatives.

With respect to health care, Yen sought the advice of the PUMC and John Grant, and to assure medical and nursing personnel for an intended health component, he spent time trying to motivate its students to work with the MEM after graduation. One evening in 1929, a small group of students gathered in the E ward of the hospital to hear Yen speak.

He opened by asserting that people are the foundation of a nation, and that national stability is dependent on their well-being. China's stability, he asserted, was threatened by the condition of its peasantry, which suffered from four interrelated problems: ignorance, poverty, poor health, and lack of public spirit. At Dingxian, he went on to say, the MEM was using an experimental approach to try to remedy these problems, based on a four-pronged, integrated approach. This entailed the development of an educational system to combat ignorance, the introduction of modern agricultural methods to alleviate poverty, the diffusion of scientific knowledge in medicine and public health to deter illness and disease, and reform in the political system to foster a spirit of public service. The research results of this social laboratory, he suggested, would be of great value to China's overall task of rural reconstruction.

Yen was a strong believer in his own movement and a persuasive speaker, and over the years he recruited six PUMC graduates in medicine and four in nursing to form a nucleus of technical personnel for the MEM Department of Health. "Sacrifice," he said, "is often needed to start something uncommon," and for the work at Dingxian, he cautioned, "You need the mind of a scientist and the heart of a missionary." John Grant was instrumental in ensuring him technical persons of high caliber, selected in accordance with criteria Yen himself established: competence, creativity, commitment, and character.

Dr. Yao Xunyuan, a PUMC graduate of the class of 1925, was appointed as first Director of the Department of Rural Health of the MEM in 1928, apparently recommended by several friends of Yen and agreed to by Grant. Yao fit the post well in that he himself was a man of rural origin, an unusual background for a PUMC graduate. As a result of his premedical schooling under the missionaries and work as a staff associate in a missionary hospital at Baodang, however, he had unconsciously absorbed a conventional, hospital-centered approach to medicine. Naturally, therefore, his plan was to undertake some general clinical work in the town and build a small district hospital. Construction of the hospital was underwritten by the Milbank Memorial Fund, but within two years of his appointment, Yao received a fellowship for advanced public health study abroad and left the MEM.

Shortly after returning from my own graduate training in the United States and Europe, Yen and Grant offered his position to me and I accepted with alacrity. I thought that the health project in itself was quite insignificant. If the model could be used for training, however, I felt that its impact on rural inhabitants could be very great. I was convinced that this could be done, that Dingxian could be developed as a rural health training station, just as the Peking First Health Station had been developed as an urban site. As for Grant, although he wanted field training posts in both rural and urban settings, he was less sanguine than I about the prospects at Dingxian. Ultimately, however, he and Yen agreed to the attempt.

As it turned out, organization of the training programs proceeded rapidly, and over the nearly six years we were in operation, we were able to provide many types of training to many sorts of health worker. We began to train village health workers almost immediately. Shortly thereafter, we added special instruction for secondary medical school graduates employed in our subdistrict health stations. In time, too, we developed an on-site rural health training facility, where we provided PUMC medical and nursing students an opportunity to practice what they learned in the classroom. To facilitate my leadership of this latter program, I was appointed to the faculty of the PUMC School of Public Health, serving concurrently in that capacity and as Director of the MEM Department of Public Health. By the time the Sino-Japanese War began in 1937, forcing us to close down, I had been teaching for some six years and held an appointment as an associate professor.

THE DINGXIAN MODEL OF COMMUNITY
MEDICINE

The interlude at Dingxian, spanning the period from January 1932 to July 1937, was a milestone in my professional life, the opening phase of a career in public health work that has continued for well over fifty years. In practical terms, the experience marked the beginning of a lifelong quest for the best means of diffusing scientific medicine within China's rural population, which more than fifty years ago was so strikingly similar to that of many developing countries today.

The work put me in contact with a great diversity of people, ranging from peasant farmers to international health specialists, yielding new understanding and appreciation of their concerns. It exposed me to a great diversity of problems, old and new, and tested my ingenuity in trying to solve them. It also provided experience that enabled me to clarify and define many of the central points in my thinking about community medicine, public health, and medical education.

Our country has a history of many millennia. But the systematic health organization developed at Dingxian was the first that had ever existed in China, bringing the benefits of modern medical care to an agricultural majority that until then had had to rely solely on indigenous beliefs and practice for medical relief.

Dingxian was barren. Its people cultivated barely enough crops to live on: corn, millet, cabbage, and turnips. These items constituted the basis of their diet, which was supplemented by a little meat. The district (the equivalent of "county" in the postrevolutionary administrative system) had no modern manufacturing enterprises whatsoever, and the only marketable commodities locally produced were a number of eye medications.

The district government supported one normal school, located in Dingxian itself, and a few primary schools. Heavy carts and donkeys, the chief means of transportation, carved deep grooves and dents into the muddy roads. A few people owned bicycles, and a ricksha could be rented.

The houses were fashioned from mud. Each room usually had only one window, so that the interiors were dark. The peasants slept on mud beds (*kang*), warmed in winter by weeds burned beneath the surface. Coal was available only for cooking. Oil lamps supplied such artificial lighting as there was. Kerosene, which was imported, was far too costly. Electricity was available only within the city limits of Dingxian.

Personally and professionally, it was very difficult for medical and nursing personnel who came from a large metropolitan city to adapt to such conditions. By that time, I had been marrried for several years, and when my family joined me we shared a house with another family, occupying three rooms all told. There were six of us, including my wife's elderly mother, using these quarters. Our sources of pleasure lay chiefly in contemplating the results of our hard work and in receiving visitors from other places.

I still remember very clearly the day—January 16, 1932, when I actually set off from Beijing for Dingxian with a group of staff members of the MEM. We left from the West Railroad Station in Beijing. By the time we arrived, there were no seats left, but someone found me a place to sit on the floor of the train. We stopped at many places along the way, and it took almost twelve hours to cover fewer than 100 miles. On arriving, we rode by mulecart over the one narrow road leading into the town.

Arrangements called for me to stay temporarily with Dr. Qu Junan, who headed the Department of Education. This was a welcome interlude, for Dr. Qu was a brilliant young intellectual, with a Ph.D. in philosophy from Harvard University. Before joining the MEM, he had taught at Yenching University.

THE BEGINNING: DEVELOPING AN INFORMATION BASE

A research group affiliated with Jin Ling University had undertaken an ongoing socioeconomic survey project in Dingxian, begun eight years earlier, and the first task I set myself, after getting my bearings, was to seek out its director, Dr. Li Jinghan. I wanted to learn as much as possible about conditions in the district.

The survey reports provided useful information on population, income, and traditional medical practice. They indicated that there was a total of 400,000 inhabitants, distributed in the town of Dingxian, various outlying market towns, and a multiplicity of surrounding villages. Annual per capita income was yuan 30—at that time the exchange rate was about Y1 = U.S.$.50. That income would provide only a bare subsistence diet for one person, mainly cereals.

The survey material also provided a certain amount of data on health and medical care, but we needed a great deal more. Yen and others of the MEM leadership were a bit skeptical about my intention to organize a local health survey, as the notion of making a field survey as the basis for formulating a health plan had no precedent.

In this particular survey we selected a sample population of about 45,000 persons. A priority interest was to establish the causes of illness and death in the district so as to determine roughly what proportion of such incidents might be prevented within the limits of medical knowledge at that time.

The results showed crude birth and death rates of 40.1 per 1,000 population and 32.1 per 1,000 population, respectively, and an infant mortality rate of 199 per 1,000 live births. Communicable diseases were responsible for much, if not most, of the illness. Among children under six years of age, diarrhea and dysentery were major causes of death. Tetanus neonatorum, formerly known as "four-to-six-day fever," however, was the leading cause of death among infants, explained in large part by the local custom of dressing the umbilical cord with mud. Besides infant diarrhea and dysentery, scarlet fever, typhoid fever, tuberculosis, measles, and smallpox were also commonplace. Analysis revealed that out of 2,032 deaths reported, 37 percent may have been entirely preventable; 32 percent more arose from conditions that could be treated successfully if reached early. While these figures were in no sense absolutely reliable, because of the uncertainty of the diagnosis, they nevertheless made it very clear that our first responsibility was to prevent communicable and infectious disease.

Another survey that I designed, covering health conditions in the schools, showed that nearly 10 percent of the children were regularly absent from classes. The reason given most frequently was "working at home." Cited next most often was "illness." Conjunctivitis and trachoma, headaches, skin diseases (i.e., scabies and pyogenic infections), sore throat, and abdominal pain—usually caused by roundworms—were the most common complaints of the absent children. Most of these conditions could have been prevented.

However tentative, the statistics clearly revealed the consequences of the lack of modern medical care and lack of knowledge about infectious diseases and how they are spread. The Adult People's Schools were teaching some hygiene, but it was important for all the villagers to know a great deal more about the causes of illness and disease. Hence I saw that, in addition to the need to establish medical facilities, the health work of experimentation must be begun quickly and be closely integrated with the educational aspects of the MEM program.

The survey revealed that the medical care available to this community was nothing other than treatment dispensed by traditional practitioners. These practitioners on whom the villagers relied had little in common with the scholar-physicians I had known in the cities. With an occasional exception, they were simply ordinary farmers who sold herbs as a sideline. They had had no special medical training and could not even read a pulse. Many were illiterate.

Even these village practitioners were not uniformly available. In fact, one-third of the district's 446 practitioners and 256 herb stores were located in a single subdistrict, whereas nearly half of the subdistricts had neither. The remaining subdistricts had anywhere from 30 to 85 practitioners and 25 to 70 herb stores.

In thinking about the quantitative and qualitative aspects of available medical care and how they could be improved, I knew that the establishment of a modern hospital, or even a series of clinics, in itself, would not remedy this situation. The only system that would have any real value was one that would extend down into the villages and improve the level of health consciousness among their inhabitants.

It was clear that in considering any solution, economic constraints would have to be constantly borne in mind. Few of the practitioners charged fees, although they did expect a compensatory gift of some sort from the patient. In actual cash outlay, villagers were spending an average of Y0.30 per capita annually on medical relief, mostly for drugs. What could possibly be accomplished on such a small amount? Expended on an individual basis, it amounted to practically nothing; however, if it were used collectively, perhaps something could be done with it.

Even with its resources pooled, no village could support a modern physician. It could not even support a nurse. Assuming an average of 100 families per village, averaging five persons each, the combined sum of available resources was only Y150. Nurses at that time were earning double that amount. An inventive solution had to be found.

Developing the Methodology

Our survey had provided us with data on health problems and socioeconomic conditions in the district. The next step was to plan a system of health care services for the inhabitants. This required considerable thought and creativity, since there was no forerunner of any kind on which we might model ourselves. I had no idea what might or might not be practical; thus, our ideas evolved as we went along.

Thinking through the development of a health program, however, I concluded that there were at least four premises on which our system should be based: it must be grounded in the village—the basic administrative unit of the district, its cost must be in accordance with the economic resources of the village, its basic personnel must come from the village, and its proper functioning must be the responsibility of the village leadership.

An Integrated Village-Based System

For purposes of administration, rural districts at that time were divided into subdistricts, and these, in turn, into villages. The subdistricts were made up of 40 to 100 villages. Only a minority of the inhabitants of any district were found in the district center or in one of its other market towns. The majority lived in rural villages. These links to each other and to the district center were slight, for travel was difficult and roads were few. Under such circumstances, a hospital- or clinic-centered approach to health care such as that used in urban China had little to recommend it. Our system had to reach everyone, not just the fortunate few in the towns. Nor were mobile clinics a practical solution for several reasons, including the inaccessibility of many villages to road traffic.

The solution I reached in time was a rural health organization that provided three levels of service built on the resources of the three administrative units: district, subdistrict, and village. The accent on integration in this structure cannot be overstressed. Units at each level in the system were supervised and supported by those at the one above, and effective interrelationships among the various parts were crucial to the effective functioning of the whole. The village nevertheless was the basic unit.

Economic Feasibility

Another premise on which the Dingxian model was based lay in the realm of economics. As already mentioned, I felt it was crucial that the village be able to financially support whatever services were to be provided at that level. Poor as the villagers were, there was no use in developing a system of health service that was inconsistent with their own resources. Commendable as such a system might be in other terms, its economic foundations were impossibly fragile. When outside aid was withdrawn, it would collapse.

The Use of Village Health Workers

My idea of using ordinary, lay people as the basic personnel of the system of rural health service seemed appropriate for essentially three reasons. First, assuming that a few villagers could be trained to undertake some preventive measures and to motivate the entire community to seek and maintain a cleaner, more sanitary environment, sources of infection could be reduced. With a lessening of illness, such skilled and technically trained personnel as were available to the system could be used to better advantage.

Second, if a few villagers could be trained to offer leadership in prevention, they could also be taught to provide initial care in emergencies or relief in simple cases, and their skill at this level could be trusted.

The post-1958 expansion of rural services in China vaulted the term "barefoot doctor" into the global lexicon, leaving many outsiders with the impression that village practitioners represented something entirely new in rural health care delivery. Actually, however, the idea of village-based lay health workers originated neither at Dingxian nor in the postliberation period. Since time immemorial, Chinese villagers had been seeking medical counsel and obtaining their medication from other villagers whose knowledge of medicine was only slightly greater than their own.

Third, it seemed theoretically plausible to use villagers—who lacked advanced technical knowledge—as the primary health workers: they were already there, and they were apt to remain there. Whereas an outsider accustomed to more amenities and less isolation might well be reluctant to suffer the hardship of village life for very long, the inhabitants were accustomed to the local conditions and were bound to their communities by kinship and other ties. Villagers who were trusted by their fellow villagers, moreover, would have an advantage over outsiders, who would have to spend precious time demonstrating their reliability.

Community Responsibility

Finally, it was our intention that, in our system, medical knowledge would filter downward, through various training programs, while medical cases would be referred upward, according to increasing complexity of condition. Success depended on the personnel at each level performing their assigned functions and performing only those functions assigned to them, or certainly in any case, nothing for which they were not trained. So those at the base level could make or break the entire system.

We knew of other rural health systems using village health personnel that had failed because insufficient attention had been given to selection, training, and supervision of such workers. Inadequate supervision could lead to any one of several unwanted outcomes. Crucial measures of prevention could be neglected. Individual patients could suffer when health workers without special expertise tried to minister beyond their capacities, or individual practitioners might begin trying to charge fees. We certainly did not want our village health workers to try to practice medicine on their own, nor did we want them to extract fees from the patients.

Such an approach would have destroyed our whole intention to make medical relief available to the entire community on a shared-cost basis. We were trying to move toward state medicine, and in the meantime we were trying to develop cooperation between the village authorities and higher officials to launch a public-supported system of medical relief that would eliminate the great economic wastage of unnecessary illness and death. I had been interested in state medicine since my student days and had written several articles on the subject for *The Binying Weekly*.

China at that time was not ready for socialized medicine, however. So in Dingxian, for the time being, we were trying to implant habits of cooperation for community welfare and to recruit volunteer labor to take preventive measures and give first aid relief. At the subdistrict health stations, where a physician was in attendance, we charged a fee that amounted to the equivalent of U.S. $0.01 or less.

The use of unpaid and only briefly trained village farmers as our basic personnel made the matter of their supervision all the more important. To maintain the confidence of the people, the health worker needed constant technical assistance and supervision. So we arranged for regular weekly exchanges between the health workers and the subdistrict physician. The health workers were in no way to be independent functionaries, acting on their own judgment and authority. Precisely the opposite; they were to be closely supervised and supported all the time. To ensure that these workers lived up to the responsibilities of the position, we made them accountable to the most powerful community organization in the village, the Alumni Associations of the Adult People's Schools. If a worker needed to be replaced for one reason or another, the Alumni Association had the authority to do so. These arrangements were of absolutely critical importance to the proper functioning of the system.

The worker needed not only supervision but also support and appreciation, which we hoped would be forthcoming from the collective membership of the Alumni Association as well as the community. Without appropriate recognition and appreciation, the morale of the village health workers, who were, after all, contributing their services free of charge, would be apt to slip. This was a great risk, because unless prevention was maintained on a continuing basis, our whole rural health effort would have very little long-term impact.

Persons examining the model of community medicine developed at Dingxian should consider it from the standpoint that it was, in fact, a community-based system, rather than that it used lay personnel (village health workers) as assistants within that system. The important points were not that the community-based system used voluntary village health workers for certain tasks but rather that village health workers constituted the lowest tier of a health maintenance system whose effective functioning began with them, and that their performance was monitored by a strong community organization responsible to ensure that quality was maintained.

It was economically unfeasible, and would remain so for many decades, for the average village to support a qualified physician or nurse, even if sufficient numbers of such personnel were available, which they were not. Yet if we were unable to reach the villages, we would have made little progress in the application of scientific medicine to improve rural health. Our solution, therefore, was to make the villagers themselves aware of the problems and arouse their sense of community responsibility and their motivation to work on the problem. That was the philosophy underlying the Dingxian model of community medicine.

The model, we fully realized, was based on the assumption of effective cooperation and collaboration of technical and nontechnical personnel. These would eventually include village health workers, to whom we gave brief training; midwives and nurses with more extensive degrees of local training; young graduates of provincial medical schools, who had completed a regular six-year medical curriculum; and physicians, graduate nurses, and students from the PUMC, who had received training on a par with that of the most advanced universities in the West. At the outset no one who was responsible for the entire area, including myself, could be absolutely certain how well the system would work.

ORGANIZATIONAL BASIS

Two steps in building the unprecedented system of organized health services in Dingxian had now been completed. We had collected the necessary epidemiological data and had decided on the key elements of our plan. We were now ready for the next step, development of the various levels of the three-tiered structure and of the linkages between the levels.

We went about this in short order, developing an organization at the apex of which was a district health center, encompassing administrative offices, a fifty-bed hospital, a laboratory, and classrooms for training. Below the district center were the various subdistrict health stations and below that, the village health workers. (A flowchart of this system is shown in fig. 1.) The system expanded quite rapidly. We began in 1932 with a district health center and two subdistrict health stations serving thirteen villages. By 1934, there were, besides the district health center, seven subdistrict health stations, serving more than seventy-five villages.

We put a great deal of thought into the selection, training, and supervision of the lay personnel who constituted the foundation of our system. We knew that the village worker concept had been tried in India, but had failed to take root there, perhaps because the village health workers had been selected by the physicians in charge of the program rather than by a peer group within the village.

In this context, I turned to the Alumni Associations of the Adult People's Schools of the MEM. The People's Schools not only gave their students basic competency in reading and writing but also tried to change their fundamental attitudes and values by imbuing in them self-reliance and community solidarity. The impetus for social change through self-effort was carried on through the Alumni Associations, whose members were spearheading the organization of agricultural cooperatives and other means of socioeconomic improvement. The basic philosophy of the MEM emphasized a correlated program of reconstruction. By training and this perspective, therefore, the members of the Alumni Association were eminently qualified to undertake a constructive project in health.

As far as the selection of village health workers for our program was concerned, my idea was to rely on the judgment of the Alumni Associations, assuming that they would choose whomever they regarded as most trustworthy and reliable. So our village health workers were elected to their positions by fellow members of these associations. With a few exceptions in villages where the organization itself was weak, the results were excellent. Our workers were generally hardworking, honest, and public-spirited.

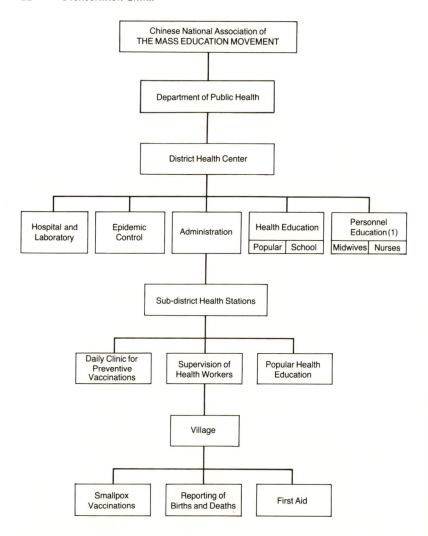

1. The rural health training site had not yet been organized.

Fig. 1. Organization of the Health System, Dingxian, 1933.

As to the scope of their responsibilities, after careful consideration, we concluded that these should be limited to the prevention of disease and the provision of simple medical relief measures. Training, however limited, could prepare the health workers for these tasks. Emphatically, however, it could not prepare them to make accurate diagnoses of other than the simplest complaints.

It was a cardinal principle in our system that the health worker should never act, or be called on to act, as a physician. The worker's three tasks, as we envisioned them, were to record births and deaths in the village, to vaccinate the community against small-pox, and to render simple treatments from the contents of a first aid box that contained a few essential and nonhazardous items. Those contents included, for example, aspirin, soda mint, oint-ment for the treatment of trachoma, a disinfectant, and bandages. With these few simple items the health worker could not commit serious errors and might be able to alleviate much unnecessary physical discomfort.

Prevention was in our minds as well. Properly trained, the worker could prevent serious conditions from developing and could refer patients upward in the system to, and through, the physician at the subdistrict health station. With physicians and students from the PUMC serving in the district health center, this put the simplest villager in a direct line of access to the best scien-tific medical knowledge in the country.

Health workers would perform their duties on a voluntary, nonre-munerative basis. We had no intention of building a new profession, nor, more importantly, of creating competitive pressure on tradi-tional practitioners. The health workers would continue to derive their income from farming and would receive no direct remunera-tion for their efforts. For now, their reward would have to be essen-tially spiritual, although perhaps in time some recompensation might be arranged for their leadership in prevention.

Village workers were in regular contact with the provincial medi-cal school graduates who served as physicians and administrative heads of the subdistrict health stations. In fact, although the station physician provided treatment to certain types of patient, the train-ing of the village health workers was the physician's first duty. This required that the physician visit the villages at regular inter-vals, and that the workers attend training sessions at the health station once a week.

Worker attitudes tended to reflect the varying attitudes and abili-ties of the health station physicians. Those physicians who were enthusiastic, took an obvious interest in what the workers were doing, and exhibited a reasonable level of competence in diagnosis and treatment earned the confidence and respect of the village health workers, who saw them as teachers, able to deal with problems they themselves could not handle.

The provincial medical school graduates were unprepared for many of the situations they encountered in both practice and teaching. Therefore, we had to supplement their education with formal instruction in vital statistics, epidemiology, and other subjects. Nevertheless, with proper supervision and help from the district health center, in spite of their inadequate foundation, most proved to be quite effective, and certainly they were able to do far more than could have been expected of a physician working entirely alone. They offered medical care at a far more skilled level than village health workers were able to provide, especially after completing the continuing education courses that were offered at the district center. Fortunately, only a few exhibited indifference to their villager patients and clearly expressed their preference for working in an urban area.

As mentioned previously, we began in 1932 with two subdistrict health stations, each staffed by a physician and a trained lay worker. Both the physician and the aide received a small salary. Later on we added a nurse to the staff of those stations that undertook school health activities. Equipment was simple, but asepsis and general cleanliness were always emphasized. The minimum setup in these stations provided the crucial link between the basic services of the village and the relatively specialized service of the district health center.

Each station was situated in a market town, which had its own subdistrict administration and one or more higher primary schools. We chose the station sites in accordance with one or the other of the two patterns of population distribution prevailing in North China at that time. One served a fairly broad area containing a few large villages separated by considerable distances. The other served a relatively small area with many small villages, separated by only short distances. Areas typified by this latter distribution pattern were usually poorer than those with a few large villages. Within a short time, the number had increased to four, including, besides the two MEM-supported units, two others financed by the local authorities.

Responsibility at the top of the system rested with the district health center, which was expected to coordinate and supplement all the activities of the subordinate agencies. The center trained the provincial medical school graduates and other local health personnel, conducted studies of special health problems, and prepared and distributed educational materials.

Additionally, the district health center operated a 50-bed hospital, whose standards were maintained at the highest possible level, while the cost of equipment and supplies was intentionally kept as low as possible. For example, patient beds were simple frame structures covered with locally produced sheets. The operating tables, also locally made, were constructed at one-sixth the price of imported tables used elsewhere. A laboratory attached to the hospital was equipped to perform routine work related to district health programs, and its staff occasionally conducted outside investigations.

From time to time, the center engaged in special projects, such as devising control measures during a cholera epidemic in 1932. Dingxian civic leaders, at the recommendation of the center, established a control committee that included, besides the magistrate, the heads of the Bureaus of Police, Education, Finance, and Public Works, several prominent tradespeople and some MEM staff members. The committee distributed wall posters, telling people how to avoid infection and urging them to be inoculated. Special police were employed to comb the countryside, looking for victims, whom they urged to seek hospitalization in the district center institution, which at that time had been in operation for less than a month. Not a single death occurred among the forty-five persons who were hospitalized with cholera. The special police supervised the disinfection of wells—which, we were told by authorities later, it was almost impossible to do in many other parts of the country because the people refused to allow it. Our villagers, by contrast, had already had some health education and understood the need. Eventually, people from neighboring areas came to us, begging for help with disinfection of their wells.

Only highly trained personnel could capably carry out the functions of the district center, so the best-educated nurses, technicians, and midwives available to us were assigned there. The project was fortunate in that these individuals were able to provide exactly the right type of leadership, without which no organized practice could succeed. Their energy, confidence, and personalities influenced the outlook of those at other levels, determining to a great extent the quality of the overall effort.

Effective communication among the three levels, in fact, was vital to proper functioning. District-level physicians met regularly with those at the subdistrict level, who, in turn, met regularly with the village workers. Through this and other integrative features, the three components of the system operated a mutually supportive network, and their joint effort represented the best form of practice that could be arranged under extremely difficult conditions.

Mapping out all the foregoing matters had been a complex and difficult task. Our reward came when the Dingxian model proved its effectiveness and we were able to gradually expand its activities, and when the central government selected it as the prototype for other district governments to follow in developing their health systems.

FIELD ACTIVITIES

Once we had implemented and staffed our organization, we launched a wide variety of field activities. From 1932 to 1935 we emphasized experimentation in refining these various activities to ensure that the principles and methods of our work would be suitable for adaptation elsewhere. Then in 1935 we were ready to move from the experimental and demonstration phase of our work to that of training.

Collection of Vital Statistics

In the experimental areas where we had already established the three-tiered infrastructure, with village health workers trained and working, we were able to keep a reliable register of vital statistics. By 1934, the number of village health workers had increased to eighty, and the number of villages in the register had tripled from our starting point. The total population in the registration area was 103,087, almost one-fourth of the district's population. Births and deaths went unreported still in other parts of the district, but in this closely controlled area, supervised by an inspector, the registration was relatively complete. The system of registering births and deaths had no counterpart elsewhere in China at that time.

Our 1934 figures for the controlled area, where we were fairly certain of the data, give an indication of important health problems. The reported rate of infant mortality was 185.2 per 1,000 live births; deaths among persons under five years of age, as a percent of all deaths, amounted to 44.5 percent, in part because of epidemics in that year from both dysentery and scarlet fever. The death rate due to dysentery was 2.3 per 1,000. Other leading causes of death included scarlet fever, pulmonary tuberculosis, tetanus neonatorum, and *kala azar*—a tropical fever transmitted by sandflies. Specific death rates from these causes were respectively 653, 178, 73, and 42 per 100,000 population. The death rate among children under two years of age from diarrhea and enteritis was 200 per 100,000. While these figures reflected a lamentably low health level, we were making progress. The rates of puerperal sepsis, tetanus neonatorum, and problems related to childbirth and early infancy in general were declining.

Provision of Medical Relief

By 1935, three years after the Dingxian experiment had begun, its various agencies were providing an impressive volume of medical relief. In that year, the hospital admitted 600 patients, providing a total of over 10,000 days of hospital care. Staff physicians performed more than 260 operations without losing a patient, and they made nearly 200 outside calls. Subdistrict stations treated more than 65,000 persons, of whom 15,000 were new patients, and village health workers administered nearly 140,000 first aid treatments.

From the standpoint of quality, there was, of course, no absolute standard; however, the general impression of the work of village health workers was that it was remarkably satisfactory. The work of the subdistrict health physicians varied in quality, reflecting variations in aptitude and training. On the whole, however, the training these physicians had received in provincial medical schools was so poor that simple diagnostic procedures became somewhat unreliable in their hands, and asepsis and cleanliness often were neglected. We tried to remedy these deficiencies as we went along, but eventually this proved futile and we had to organize further formal coursework for them.

Furtherance of Sanitation

The value of potable water supplies and appropriate sanitation in disease prevention is immeasurable, but regrettably, rural sanitary engineering was an unexplored field at that time, and we could find no one professionally trained to help us. Nevertheless, we did our best with the limited possibilities at hand.

For example, we decreased contamination in village wells by making two changes. First, we had the farmers raise the level of the mouths of the wells so as to prevent surface water pollutants from draining down into the cavities. Second, we replaced individual family buckets with a common bucket, hung permanently on a hook at the top of the well. Because that bucket never came into contact with contamination from the ground, as had the buckets that family members brought and set down in the adjacent area while waiting their turns to draw water, this too, decreased pollution to an extent. Compared with the enormous need, our efforts were marginal, but every little bit helped.

Bathing facilities in the village had been nonexistent. It was commonly said at that time that villagers bathed or were bathed only three times in a lifetime: at birth, at marriage, and at death. So we built some communal bathhouses. Our three bathhouses opened 121 times that year, and we noted that 8,500 baths were taken. The schoolchildren and village health workers bathed free of charge; others paid Yo.01 each. This may sound primitive, but it was really an innovation in community life. It was also of great importance in rural China at that time, not for aesthetic reasons alone, but because skin infections, which could be prevented by frequent bathing, were so commonplace.

Control of Communicable Diseases

At that time (mid-1930s), smallpox was still prevalent. Attempts had been made in many parts of the country to prevent its spread by vaccination programs. These failed in most instances because authorities were unable to reach every family, and even among those whom they reached, the issue of who was most at risk by virtue of age was neglected. In Dingxian, however, this was not a question. We could reach a very high percentage of the population at risk, and we got to the children who most needed it; thus, we were able to go a long way in controlling the disease. In time, when smallpox broke out in neighboring areas, it did not appear in ours.

Vaccination against cholera was another success story. In 1934 North China as a whole suffered an epidemic of cholera, but Dingxian and surrounding areas had only a few cases, and even those were successfully treated in our hospital.

Health Education

The Department of Rural Health provided health education for all primary-school children and for various adult groups, reflecting the strong belief of its director that general medical work must always be correlated with educational work. We began with the children for several reasons. They were at a receptive, impressionable age when new habits can be formed easily. They attended school for a two-year period at least, which gave us an opportunity to reinforce the teaching over an extended period. Moreover, they could serve as a conduit through which we could indirectly teach something to the older generation.

For our health education program we relied heavily on the primary-school teachers and the school nurse. First, however, we had to teach the teachers. As it was, students in the normal schools received an education heavily weighted toward the theoretical side, emphasizing teaching principles and techniques of administration, and often neglecting practical subject material. We had to convince the teachers both that teaching hygiene was worthwhile and that it was their responsibility. Next, we arranged for a special nurse to prepare a series of textbooks on the subject. To correlate with the lessons, we issued earthenware spitoons, washbasins, and individual drinking cups to be distributed to the children.

The importance of potable water received special emphasis; with the help of village health workers, we constructed many new school wells or disinfected existing ones, or made arrangement to supply boiled water where neither of these measures could be accomplished. We also built latrines.

A nurse visited each school on a regular weekly basis, treating the children for various ear and eye conditions and ringworm of the scalp and referring those with dental problems to a special clinic. Contents of a school first aid box were available to the nurse; such boxes had been supplied at a minimal cost through the MEM. Schools replenished the contents at their own expense, amounting to less than Y1.00 annually.

For the adults, I personally revised *The One Thousand Characters* text of the Adult People's Schools to include eight complete lessons and four references to health in the four-months course. Also, the district health center held an annual health exhibit during Chinese New Year, when thousands of villagers flocked to Dingxian. Staff members distributed health literature and demonstrated proper ways of bathing and feeding children.

Improvement of Maternal and Child Health

Progress in the realm of maternal and child health was impeded by prevailing social attitudes and economic conditions. Maternal welfare was not a subject that elicited much interest or concern in the village. In the rare instances when a case did become an issue, the outcome was often adverse. For example, some pregnant young wives wanted very much to deliver in the district health center under the care of a qualified midwife but were effectively discouraged from doing so by their mothers-in-law, whose ideas carried great weight in the family, and who thought delivery should take place at home.

Our program also included family planning, for which any forward-looking social program should provide. Villagers at that time believed that there was no way of limiting the number of children they might produce. We were among the first, if not *the* first, group to make family planning services available.

We might have achieved more had it not been for an entangled web of economic circumstances and traditional social values that stood in the way. Among the obstacles was the strong village preference for large families. Sons were especially desired because they were expected to carry on the family line and to increase the prosperity of the family; moreover, there was always an outside chance that a son might become famous and add luster to the family name. Another major impediment was the lack of any tested and safe means of contraception, one sufficiently simple and inexpensive for extensive use under rural conditions.

The Department of Health did undertake some successful programs. Seeking to reduce the high rate of infant mortality, we enrolled a number of mothers in short classes for housewives, made many pre- and postnatal visits at home, and persuaded a continually growing number of women to deliver their babies at the district center under qualified care.

In other areas, such as midwifery, we encountered difficulties and made mistakes. Sometimes the solution to a particular problem was so elusive that we were almost inclined to abandon the issue. At that time, child delivery was still in the hands of ignorant old women. So, at first, we brought in a specially trained young midwife, with an experienced physician of obstetrics to back her up.

The villagers would not accept an outsider of only twenty-five years of age as a trustworthy person, however. Moreover, there were so few abnormal labor cases that the back-up physician was a luxury.

So we attempted to retrain the old traditional midwives. This turned out to be difficult for many reasons. Because these midwives were unable to read and write, special instructional materials had to be prepared. Furthermore, the traditional midwives resented the young, unmarried woman we selected as the trainer. She had had advanced training, and they had not. She was relatively well educated, and they were illiterate. Nevertheless, they regarded her as an inexperienced upstart and demonstrated a good deal of jealousy. In any event, we learned that it was very difficult to correct their lifetime habits, even to enforce the practice of cleanliness.

Eventually, rather than retraining the old midwives, we selected and trained one of their younger relatives, who, as a member of their own family, would receive the older woman's support in her new role. This approach also eliminated the problem of jealousy. We thought that at last we had made an encouraging start. After a time, however, we found that this was impractical; the young woman was usually too busy to fulfill the responsibilities of this extra and irregular work.

This lurching back and forth on such an urgent problem as the need for qualified midwifery was very frustrating, but experience has reinforced our belief that there is no easy solution to this question. Changing attitudes in this area may take more than one generation.

INSTRUCTIONAL ACTIVITIES

By 1935, in just a few short years, our field activities had expanded enormously and, despite many difficulties, we were rendering a great deal of help to the villagers. In relation to these activities, we had organized four different types of training or continuing education. We were now prepared to shift our focus from the various clinical and health education activities to the training programs, whose students included both our own staff members and medical and nursing undergraduates at other institutions.

Our key training program was that provided to the village health workers. The preparation of rudimentarily educated villagers to serve as basic personnel in a three-tiered integrated rural health system had been an exceptional challenge. No one in our country had even conceived of such a program at that time.

After some discussion, the MEM leadership had agreed with my general plan to provide ten days of training to each worker. I proposed that a group should meet for instruction at some suitable central point, such as a primary school or a subdistrict health station, that each student could reach on foot within an hour or so. This would obviate the expense of overnight accommodations. Classes would meet daily on a regular basis.

The Alumni Association would play a sustentative role. It would bear the cost of a free noon meal to each volunteer. More importantly, after training was completed, the association was expected to give continuous moral support to the volunteer so as to nurture continuing interest in the work. Arrangements for words of praise from the magistrate and a small annual "bonus" that could be graded according to definite standards of achievement, for example, provided ample incentive.

Some MEM spokespersons had been skeptical about the proposed length of the training session, thinking that ten days was too short. Experience proved that this was a good decision, however. To be sure, we wanted to avoid at all costs giving the impression that we were training "doctors." In any case, the intent of our training was not so much to convey factual information as it was to institute a good working relationship between the student and the health station physician who would serve as that student's supervi-

sor. We believed in accenting supervised practice rather than classroom explanations as the primary learning method.

As director of the department, I felt that I should train at least
the first group of health workers before passing the task along to
the subdistrict health station physicians, not because I had experience but because I wanted to experiment to find the best means of
doing it. Choices as to what to emphasize had to be made and a
syllabus prepared.

In retrospect, it seemed appropriate to concentrate on certain
areas: general matters of hygiene, emphasizing cleanliness; birth
and death registry; immunization techniques; smallpox control;
and measures of prevention for trachoma and skin infections.
These choices reflected, in general, the prevailing major health
problems in the area and, in particular, the relative simplicity and
low cost of eliminating smallpox. The importance of maintaining a
vital statistics registry was evident.

The syllabus, as it evolved, contained seven lessons, to be presented within ten days or less. The first lesson covered general
health matters, focusing on infection, treatment of cuts, and use of
antiseptics and the importance of cleanliness. We discussed the
need to keep the eyes clean to avoid infection that could lead to
trachoma and the need to wash clothes to prevent lice infestation.
The second lesson, given in two parts, dealt with water supplies
and latrine construction and techniques for vaccination against
smallpox and cholera. The third lesson offered a review and individual practice in vaccination techniques. The fourth delved deeper
into the topics of cleanliness and sterilization, introduced the student to the contents of the first aid box, and addressed the dangers
of opium smoking and the hazard of carbon monoxide poisoning.
Brief remarks on the disadvantages of large families and some famil-
iarization with quinine suppositories and the metallic cervical ring
in this context were also offered. Workers were advised of the
value of soybean milk in infant feeding. The fifth lesson provided
for practice in bandaging and other first aid techniques. The sixth
offered another review, together with instructions for completing
simple birth and death forms. We recommended that symptoms of
illness be listed where the cause of death was uncertain. The final
lesson covered some clinical material and then shifted to regula-

tions concerning the use of certain medications and to procedures for referring patients to the subdistrict stations.

When I turned the training over to the subdistrict health station physicians, I was well aware that the success of the training depended not only on what was taught but also on the personality of the teacher. The instructor had an inherent advantage in that, in our cultural tradition, the teacher–pupil relationship is generally respected. Still, mutual respect and confidence must be developed on an individual basis. So we urged the physicians who trained the villagers to use simple language, avoid the use of technical terminology, and keep their expectations of the students modest.

Concerning substance, we insisted that they stress proper execution of the task at hand, rather than the acquisition of additional skills. For example, the physician as trainer was to convince the workers of the importance of filling in registration forms completely; of describing symptoms of terminal illness as accurately as possible; of giving vaccinations according to prescribed procedures; of providing additional commentary when handing out health literature; and, above all, of not making their own diagnoses, but rather sending patients to a trained physician at the subdistrict station.

In the final analysis, this phase of our training program was exceptionally successful. The syllabus proved satisfactory, the teachers capable, and the health workers reliable and responsive. Personally, I found the enthusiasm of the village workers really inspiring; they were always enthusiastic and eager to learn, they did not expect too much remuneration, and they were uniformly proud of their ability to assist their fellow villagers.

Experience quickly revealed that the subdistrict station physicians themselves needed more training. We had visualized that when the Dingxian model was adopted throughout the country, in accordance with the 1934 central government recommendation, graduates of provincial medical schools would head the subdistrict health stations, while graduates of the better medical schools would head the district health centers.

Within each of these two categories of medical school, however, there was great diversity in the quality of training from institution to institution; medical education in China at that time had no uniform standard. We had only the broadest of notions of what could be expected of an individual graduate, therefore, and in any event the training of all provincial school graduates was poor. This was apparent in the typical neglect of asepsis among the graduates and their ineptness in diagnosis. Nursing education also was deficient. Moreover, the training students received in clinical medicine and in public health even at the better medical schools was weak. Before we were willing to entrust certain responsibilities to the young physicians, therefore, it was necessary to supplement crucial gaps in their training.

In time, we organized a two-year in-service training program for physicians serving in rural subdistrict health stations. It proved satisfactory, although in developing its curriculum, we had, as in so many other instances, no experience to guide us.

The general plan called for classroom instruction during the first year, with supervised practice in the field. The second year was devoted completely to supervised field practice. This emphasis reflected a strong personal conviction, originating in experience in European and American public health schools, that postgraduate training for technically trained personnel is most effective when founded on participation in responsible activities, under supervision. Inasmuch as the field facilities in Dingxian were well developed and were directly under the control of the Department of Health, the opportunity of developing students by the academically sound technique of "learning by doing" seemed unique.

The classroom discussion component of the program was arranged on a monthly basis. At the outset, in September, there was a two-week opening session devoted to general rural problems. This was followed by regular weekly sessions over a nine-month period, with a special topic addressed each month. From October to June, these were, respectively: (1) asepsis and elementary nursing practice, (2) diagnostic techniques, (3) health education and school health, (4) training and supervision of village workers, (5) rural public health principles, (6) smallpox control, (7) sanitation, (8) rural medical relief, and (9) administrative problems in rural health practice.

Because the students constituted the crucial link between the district and village levels, implementation of rural programs was highly dependent on the ability of these students, and it was essential to prepare them well. Their reaction to the supplementary program was essentially positive, although initially many objected to being given instruction in nursing techniques. By the end of the month, however, they realized the significance of simple techniques and had developed an appreciation of the nurses' contribution. The sessions devoted to diagnosis, led by senior members of the medical staff, proved to be of special interest to the group.

Rural health nursing represented another locus of training effort. We ran two nursing education programs, one a three-year undergraduate program for young women of the district, the other a six-month program for graduate nurses—all, of course, trained in hospitals in other parts of the country. The graduate nurses were prepared for such tasks as development of school health work, collaboration in communicable disease eradication programs, and supervision of village workers and local midwives. Nothing like this program existed anywhere else in China. Through the undergraduate program, we were hoping to develop a supply of local nurses who would live and work in the area and who were familiar with the problems of rural health practice.

Ultimately, we organized the final component of our system, completing the bridge we had hoped to construct between rural and urban China, giving villagers in a remote rural district access to the most advanced scientific medical knowledge in China. From its inception the MEM had relied on the PUMC for advice and personnel in the medical field. Now we were prepared to offer a valuable resource in return, a rural health field training site.

Once the demonstration course in rural public health had been established at Dingxian, it drew undergraduate and postgraduate students not only from the PUMC but also from Shanghai Medical College and Hunan–Yale Medical College in Hunan. We devised a similar program for PUMC nursing students as well. The students came in small groups, spending anywhere from three days to four weeks with us, during which time they gained firsthand impressions of conditions in the market towns and villages of an ordinary rural district.

To emphasize the contrast with conditions of practice in urban China and to highlight the harsh realities of rural China's health and medical problems, I always used local examples, as my own public health professor had done. When the students visited the wards, they saw us using locally manufactured equipment and locally constructed facilities as best we could. Before touring the wards of the district center hospital, the students were always furnished with complete records on the patients they saw. Lectures on preventive medicine, highlighting vaccination measures and school health, were reinforced with field trips to the villages, which permitted exchanges on health matters with the local inhabitants.

While all this experience provided a stark realization of the difficulties of providing quality care under such circumstances, it also showed how challenging it could be to formulate inventive solutions to seemingly insoluble problems. Although the clerkship in rural health was rather short, most of the students seem to have been deeply impressed by it and felt that it was a highpoint of their undergraduate education in rural health.

Without an effective field organization, we could never have provided such an experience, of course, and we stressed to each group that wherever they found themselves after graduation, if they went into the public health field, they would also have to devote time and attention to administrative matters. Otherwise there could be no assurance of quality. Technological knowledge alone would not suffice; they also had to become knowledgeable about administration.

Besides giving training to students who came to us, Miss Zhang, the nurse-midwife on our staff, and I did some training on the outside, at the Hubei Provincial Medical School. She conducted a midwifery course, and I taught a regular four-hours-per-week course in public health for the medical undergraduates. These and other cooperative training and research activities added to the pressures on my time.

The training programs at Dingxian improved the quality of care being administered because the continual influx of outsiders stimulated those directly involved in the training programs to continue to improve their skills. There were broader benefits as well, for the training we provided would have been noteworthy on the basis of the number of persons we exposed to rural health problems alone. Beyond this, we felt we were paving the way for the development of medical education in relation to community needs in other parts of China as well. In that respect it was an important step toward my own personal goal of introducing scientific knowledge gradually, carefully, and continuously among the rural people.

RESIDUAL PROBLEMS

We could look back on our accomplishment at Dingxian with pride. About three years after we had begun, the Dingxian model of community medicine had demonstrated its practicability under prevailing conditions in rural areas of North China. At a minimum it had proved effective in limiting the spread of communicable disease and meeting the most urgent medical needs of villagers, while most agreed that its accomplishments went far beyond that. We had devised a model of rural health care delivery that could be implemented anywhere in our vast and diverse country, linking remote villages to the most advanced technical centers in the cities. Also, while doing so, as Robert S. K. Lim and others noted, we had demonstrated an important principle of medical education, specifically, that it is entirely possible to correlate instruction in public health and clinical medicine in a meaningful way.

Before hostilities with Japan curtailed our experimentation after 1937, we had intended, among other things, to expand our survey field to cover a larger statistical database, and, while doing so, improve the accuracy of reporting.

Also, we were quite aware that our family planning efforts needed expansion. I had already discussed my conviction that a sound family planning program was crucial to overall health improvement with Dr. Marshall Balfour, who succeeded John Grant as Far Eastern representative of the International Health Division of the Rockefeller Foundation. Few, if any, responsible government officials in China in the 1930s, however, shared my conviction; in fact, some saw no correlation at all between fewer births and improved health. Understandably, therefore, there were no family planning programs of any kind in our country at that time, either public or private. Prevailing social values and economic conditions mitigated against such programs at every turn. This problem was of a greater order of magnitude than the need to expand our sample population, therefore, and single-handedly at Dingxian, we could make only limited progress against it.

Another generalized problem that concerned us at Dingxian was how little the urban-trained medical school graduates actually knew of rural life and how inadequately their training had prepared them for dealing with the problems of the peasants, who, after all, represented the majority of our population. We had begun to address this issue by organizing our rural field training site. We all knew that this was only a start, however. As far as the entire country was concerned, it was urgent that far larger numbers of medical students be given practical experience in the application of scientific knowledge in the countryside.

Economic issues also needed attention. In particular, we had not yet really solved the question of how to remunerate the village health workers. The professional staff at Dingxian were receiving modest salaries out of general funds for the experiment, although they were received less than their peers in urban practice. The village services were to be self-supporting, however, and although the clinics received some income from miniscule patient fees, these funds could not be stretched to provide a salary for the village health workers, and we managed by asking them to volunteer, giving them a bonus and words of praise from the district magistrate at the end of the year. This worked satisfactorily enough, but it was no long-term solution.

A related issue concerned the support of the system in toto. We believed that we had devised a system well within the economic reach of the villages, given that collectively, district inhabitants had been paying about Y120,000 per year for medical service of one kind or another. The cost of our system would be less than Y40,000, or Y0.10 per person, so there was margin to spare. Nevertheless, the question remained as to how the available resources could be concentrated for collective use. Jimmy Yen and I frequently discussed the possibility that this could be accomplished under government authority; this was why relations between the MEM and the district government were becoming increasingly close. Already the Dingxian district authorities were becoming interested, and whereas they had expended practically nothing for community health in 1932, by 1935 they were pledging Y12,000 annually to the health system. It was a step toward state medicine, an idea we had been advocating since student days at the PUMC.

OBSERVATIONS OF RURAL HEALTH
PROGRAMS ABROAD

While serving as Director of the Department of Rural Health at Dingxian, I personally had many opportunities to meet and talk to other persons working in public health, community medicine, and medical education both at home and abroad. Biennial meetings of the Chinese Medical Association provided one lively forum of interchange. Other opportunities arose in discussion with guest lecturers at the PUMC, foreign and domestic visitors who came to Dingxian, and my own travel abroad. Visitors at Dingxian, for example, included Selskar Gunn of the International Health Division of the Rockefeller Foundation; Marian Yang, a Chinese national and a nurse, who had developed an innovative program at the Peking Urban Health station for retraining traditional midwives under urban conditions; and Dr. Andrija Stampar, a public health physician from Yugoslavia and highly respected figure in eastern European social medicine, whom we enjoyed especially. Both individually and collectively, these experiences taught me that a great deal of understanding and appreciation derives from free exchange of ideas among persons of various backgrounds.

My main experience in the context of international exchange during the 1930s was an extended study trip abroad in 1935, which included visits to the Soviet Union, Yugoslavia, and India. It was on Stampar's recommendation that the Ministry of Health and the League of Nations arranged for my visit to these countries. Because of the article on proteolytic enzymes that I had written as a PUMC student under Robert S. K. Lim, I traveled to the Soviet Union with a group of physiologists, who, with Lim as head, were to attend an international conference on physiology in Leningrad.

On the way to the Soviet Union, the delegation traveled by rail through Manchuko (Manchuria), which at that time was already under Japanese occupation, although open war would not break out between our two countries for two more years. The journey by train from Beijing to Moscow took ten days. At Mukden, the Japanese confined us to the train, not even allowing us to step down onto the platform. Farther north, at Harbin, we changed trains and headed for Manchouli, on the Siberian border. There I had the terrible experience of seeing a young Japanese railroad officer brutally cuff an old Chinese peasant across the face, as well as kick him violently. The old man dared not cry, and the people around him remained silent. I was indignant and ashamed, but I could not help that poor fellow.

In Moscow, official interpreters met our train. Although I was to learn Russian fifteen or so years later, I did not speak the language at that time, nor did anyone in our group. We shared a Ford taxi to our hotel with two Americans, who complained under their breaths at the slowness of the vehicle. Their English was not lost on the driver, however, who turned to the surprised passengers in the rear of the cab and remarked, for their benefit, "Nothing in the world can be done without patience."

At the hotel, several young, well-dressed, English-speaking women arranged our travel plans. They assigned me to a sparsely furnished room that I shared with Dr. Hou Zonglian, who some years hence would become dean of the Shanxi Provincial Medical College. Later I met some old friends, including an Austrian physician who had once visited Dingxian, and Hilda Yen, niece of Dr. W. W. Yen, China's ambassador to the Soviet Union, with whom she was staying. The ambassador welcomed the Chinese delegation with a banquet at the embassy. Later in Leningrad, we were entertained by the Russians as well. There we attended a large reception replete with an elaborate buffet and many vodka toasts.

Our general impressions were limited, as we were not free to stray far from the hotel. The people we observed on the surrounding streets were quite simply dressed in contrast to our hotel guides, and we saw few smiling faces. We were told that there was a thriving black market. The subway trains were clean and comfortable, and the tunnels were paved with marble and decorated with large wall paintings.

Transportation and hotel accommodations in Leningrad were better than those in Moscow. The conference of physiologists was held in the hall of a great palace built before the Revolution. Foreign Minister I. V. Molotov addressed the group. The size and scale of the conference was impressive as there were hundreds of delegates from all over the world. Disappointingly, however, there were few small group discussions. We met the over-80-year-old, world-renowned physiologist Ivan Pavlov, who walked with a cane and had little to say. Assistants demonstrated his experiments with the conditioned reflex in a small laboratory, which was simply equipped and somewhat outmoded. Nothing was mentioned of his world-famous work on gastric-juice secretions.

Local tours in Moscow and Leningrad included visits to a teaching hospital in a medical school, a tuberculosis santitarium for children, and an abortion hospital. The teaching hospital was an old, rather decrepit building. My guide, a middle-aged woman who spoke fairly good English, took me only to wards containing ten or more patients. They were not entirely clean. To my surprise, an elderly professor of gynecology commented to me privately: "No drugs. No equipment. I wish I could work in another country." At the tuberculosis sanitarium children of all ages were being treated with sunbathing and special diets. The institution itself appeared to be well managed, but nothing was mentioned about diagnostic techniques or patient recovery rates.

While it was to reverse its policy after World War II, the Soviet Union was concerned at that time about a problem of overpopulation, and Moscow alone had four hospitals devoted exclusively to performing abortions. While I was able to visit one such hospital, I was never able to learn exactly how many beds were available for this purpose. I watched one abortion being performed, an unpleasant experience in that it was done with a special long spoon and no anesthesia, and my impression was that it was quite hard on the patient. The patient made no complaint but frowned as she walked away from the surgery, disregarding other young women in the room who were laughing under their breaths, seemingly because they found her discomfort amusing.

The same interpreter accompanied me to Kiev, in the Ukraine, and thinking about the incidence of abortion, I discussed the issue with her. She was willing to talk at length on the subject, emphasizing that there was great public resistance to contraception, especially on the part of men, who were generally unwilling to use condoms. In Kolkhis, we visited a collective farm to view its nursery. There, two elderly women were caring for about twenty infants. The children were fed unpasteurized milk and there was apparently no trained medical attention available. The place was unclean and fly-infested.

Border officials permitted me to retain the many articles on health in the Soviet Union that my interpreter provided, so I was able to bring them home. In Geneva, where I met with League of Nations officials, I was asked my impressions of the visit. The Soviet Union, I answered, was ahead of many countries in practicing state medicine, but the quality of its service had to be improved.

Subsequently I visited Yugoslavia, where I found conditions to be quite different and much more interesting. Dr. Borislav Borcic, who for two years had served the Chinese Ministry of Health in an advisory capacity, had arranged for me to visit rural health care facilities in the Croatian region of the country. Accompanied by two sanitary engineers, a Mr. Petrik and a Mr. Tedorovitch, I traveled extensively through this area for three months in a motor vehicle equipped for rough terrain.

Their rural health program had two chief components, a system of small health centers and a project to improve rural water supplies. An experienced nurse administered each health center and was responsible for teaching hygiene to children and adults, stressing personal cleanliness and protection against infectious disease. She also gave some first aid treatments. The centers were quite numerous but, in contrast to village health stations in China, had no apparent link to any agency offering medical relief under a trained physician. Moreover, I saw no other evidence of any systematic effort to apply scientific medical knowledge, preventive or curative, in rural areas.

As to the provision of potable water in the rural areas, a really remarkable number of wells had been constructed. While some were rather shallow, all had been protected with a cover as well as supplied with a pump. The pumps were not the usual pressure type; rather, they had a series of metal cups, which functioned generally like windmill buckets, continuously dipping water from the well and channeling it into a pipe, from which there was a perpetual flow of fresh water. The device was much less expensive than a pressure pump and relatively easier to repair in case of damage.

These wells were distributed throughout the rural areas, providing the villagers with easy access to fairly clean drinking water. They could also use the water for washing, as it was quite abundant. There was also a minor program of school health, directed by Andrija Stampar's wife, about which I heard when I had dinner with them in their home one night.

In Zagreb, the Croatian province capital, my hosts took me to the Rockefeller Foundation–supported institute of hygiene, which, not unlike the MEM, advocated an integrated approach to the solution of rural problems. The range of interest of this institution was broader than ours, however, and its faculty and staff included, in addition to medical personnel, sanitary engineers, agronomists, and specialists in veterinary medicine. I sat in on a discussion of modern storage of livestock feed. This was quite unlike the institutes of hygiene and schools of public health that I knew of elsewhere at the time. Those I was familiar with in the United States seemed to be concerned more with theoretical knowledge and scientific research than with the practical application of scientific knowledge for the benefit of the general population. Regrettably, decades later public health professors in the West seemed to be encouraging graduate students along the same lines.

My country, I later noted, was relatively deficient in developing a potable water supply system and in implementing sanitary engineering as a major part of the public health service. Economic conditions would have made it very difficult to construct wells of the type found in Yugoslavia, however. Moreover, China had few sanitary engineers and only one small department of civil engineering at Qinghua University that concerned itself with sanitary engineering and whose cooperation, in any event, was difficult to secure on projects such as Dingxian.

The final visit of the journey, to India and Ceylon, was a disappointment. Most of the time was spent in Colombo and the surrounding regions of what is now Sri Lanka. I saw only some hookworm control clinics, where the part-time physicians failed to make careful examination of patients, and where laboratory evidence was generally lacking. The attitude of the physicians toward the poor peasants suffering from disease was quite unpleasant; for example, they reprimanded even seriously ill patients for not following directions properly.

India's vertical approach to health care disturbed me because I believe so strongly that health improvement cannot be achieved without concurrent progress in in other socioeconomic areas. A minority of Indians seemed to enjoy all the advantages of modern science in Western civilization, while the vast majority had very little; food, clothing, and shelter were critical problems. I have no firsthand knowledge of the situation at present; it may be much better.

Of all that I had seen, I was most impressed with work being done among the peasants in Yugoslavia. On the whole, I came away more certain than ever that we were on the right path of rural health experience with the Dingxian model, as it was based on working closely with the villagers in helping them solve their problems. I returned to work with heightened enthusiasm and was able to continue for two more years before the Sino-Japanese War began in 1937.

4

Medicine and Health Under Wartime Conditions

W hile the work at Dingxian had been going on, the Japanese had been pushing further into North China and along the coastal provinces. In mid-1937, open, although undeclared, war broke out between the two countries, making it impossible to continue our field training. For nearly thirteen years thereafter, China knew hardship and chaos, caused partly by Japanese aggression and partly by the corruption of the Nationalist regime, whose indifference to the concerns of the people in the end left broad segments of the population, including many intellectuals, disdainful of its leadership.

Shortly after we were compelled to discontinue the Dingxian experiment, I left Beijing to do war relief work in South China, initially joining Robert S. K. Lim in Changsha, in Hunan Province. Not long after, I was asked to lend help in my native city of Chengdu, in Sichuan Province, which was being heavily bombed by Japanese warplanes. So I returned home in May 1939.

There, aside from organizing relief for the wounded, I taught public health in two local universities and in the early 1940s, notwithstanding the ongoing conflict, in my capacity as provincial commissioner of health, organized a provincewide system of state medicine, based on the Dingxian model. The Sino-Japanese War ended in 1945, and in 1946, I was invited to Chongqing, another major city in Sichuan Province, to establish a new medical college. Once the medical college at National Chongqing University became operational, I served as its dean and as a professor in its

School of Public Health until 1952. While these experiences were of an order different from that at Dingxian, they, too, provided valuable insights that furthered my evolving views on rural health, community medicine, and medical education.

PRELIBERATION CHINA: 1937 TO 1949

Meanwhile, in the enemy-occupied heartland of China, the Guomindang and its Western allies and the Chinese Communist party (CCP) were collaborating in a show of internal unity against external danger to try to oust the Japanese. Notwithstanding a barely concealed mutual emnity, the uneasy alliance between the Guomindang and Communists was maintained throughout the war years. After Japan's surrender in 1945, the united front predictably broke apart, revealing a nation that was in fact politically divided and economically in ruins.

Support for the Guomindang had eroded widely. In the interim the CCP not only had amassed a broad base of peasant support but also had gained the allegiance of many urban intellectuals, including some medical specialists. Disillusioned by the failures and the excesses of the Guomindang, this educated group was now pinning its hopes for the country's future on the Communist leadership and the ideological commitment of that leadership to socialist principles. To them, the party commitment to the well-being of the common people seemed to proffer hope for a better country and, with it, the prospect of health protection for all.

The civil war that broke out in China after the close of the Sino-Japanese War spanned four more years and exacted a high price in lives and human suffering. Those who supported the CCP were rewarded with victory at last in 1949, however, with the flight of Chiang Kai-shek and his supporters to Taiwan Province and the proclamation of the People's Republic of China in Beijing in October of that year.

HEALTH DEVELOPMENT AND MEDICAL
EDUCATION IN SICHUAN PROVINCE

What I am able to add to an account of the Chinese experience in rural health development during the Sino-Japanese War and there-

after until 1949 is limited to what I knew through my immediate
personal experience or through personal contacts in southwestern
China. In that part of the country, which felt the impact of the
hostilities but managed to evade occupation, medical personnel
stayed in touch as best they could and functioned in their roles
wherever they found themselves.

Quite a few modern-trained physicians left their native cities in
the Japanese-controlled northern and coastal regions or the central
Yangtze River valley and resettled farther in the interior. There
they convened on several occasions at general meetings of the
Chinese Medical Association (CMA), called by its president, P.Z.
Jin. Jin, who had been elected to his office just before the war,
retained oversight of CMA affairs during this period. The meetings
in both Kunming in 1940 and Chongqing in 1943 were relatively
well attended considering that a major war was under way. Some
500 members attended the first postwar meeting, held in Nanjing,
and twenty-five papers were presented. Dr. Zhu Zhanggen was
elected to the presidency in 1947.

The Dingxian experiment, which had just begun to gain national
and international recognition, ended shortly after the incident at
the Marco Polo bridge on July 7, 1937. Japanese forces soon occupied Beijing, and it became impossible to offer systematic field
training at the Dingxian site. Many staff members left at once. A
few subdistrict personnel and village health workers remained but
by the following year operations had terminated entirely.

For the moment, my personal future remained clouded. Two
years earlier, in 1936, I had been appointed superintendent of
both the Peking First Health Station and the Dingxian Rural
Health Station. Earnings from my various posts allowed me to
provide comfortably for my family, and medical officers of the
Japanese occupational forces expressed interest in, and respect
for, my work.

Without sovereignty, however, it was useless to attempt constructive activities. Moreover, the brutality of the Japanese milita-
rists toward the defeated Chinese seemed unconscionable to me;
their behavior reignited the intense Nationalist sentiments I had
experienced as a medical student during the anti-British protests of
1925. It became impossible to remain closeted within the walls of
academe at such a time. Indignation and patriotism compelled me

to find some alternative, some way to apply my medical training on behalf of my compatriots.

So, in May 1938, at my own expense, I left Beijing in great secrecy to join Professor Robert S. K. Lim, in war relief work in South China. Lim meanwhile had been appointed director of the Chinese Red Cross, whose headquarters were at Changsha, capital of Hunan Province. My departure from Beijing was so secret that neither the medical college nor the staff of the Peking First Health Station had been informed of my intention to leave.

In a very roundabout journey, I made my way to Changsha in South China. Fang Shih-san, a returned student from Japan and a member of the PUMC Board of Trustees, had been able to secure a permit for me to travel via Tianjin and Shanghai. So I followed that route and then took an ocean liner to Hongkong and from there a plane to Changsha to join Lim.

By the time I arrived at Changsha, Japanese forces were already pushing very close to the city and Guomindang forces were retreating. The Chinese Red Cross had withdrawn farther into the interior, southwestward some 400 miles, to Guiyang, capital of Guizhou Province. Pressing on to Guizhou, I found the Chinese Red Cross there inadequately organized to work efficiently, so I had to abandon plans for useful activity through that channel.

In the same province, however, I found an opportunity for constructive action through the North China Council of Rural Reconstruction. The council had recently transferred its operations to Guizhou Province from Shandong Province, which had been one of the first areas occupied by the Japanese. Like the PUMC, the North China Council of Rural Reconstruction was a Rockefeller-supported program, but its objective was developmental rather than educational. Broadly stated, its principal goal was national reconstruction with special reference to rural problems;[1] it offered experimental training to university students in public health, agriculture, and other fields. I became head of its Health Department and acting director of its Rural Institute.

The field activities of the council were based in Dingfan District, some twenty miles from Guiyang, a rural area not unlike Dingxian. Soon after my arrival, arrangements were concluded for Dingfan to become a site for field training in community medicine for senior medical students from Guiyang Provincial Medical College, just as

PUMC and other students in North China had been sent to Dingxian. One of my students there later became dean of the School of Public Health of Kunming Medical College.

ORGANIZING WARTIME MEDICAL RELIEF

At this moment the provincial government of Sichuan was reorganized under a new secretary-general, and I was asked to return to Chengdu, the city where I had been born, to organize a medical relief program. Up to that time the government had made no provision for war victims, and such provision was badly needed. Japanese bombs were wounding and killing inhabitants of the city every day. My father, who was still living at the time, urged me to return home.

Although I was reluctant to return for several reasons, I finally decided to do so, compelled by the dire need of the local inhabitants. My hesitation arose partly from reluctance to leave newly assumed responsibilities with the North China Council of Rural Reconstruction and partly from my hesitation to undertake a program that was to receive practically nothing in the way of support. Even with the best financing, it would have been difficult enough to organize and run such a program. But I was to be given only Y3,000 to start operations, the equivalent of the cost of 800 to 1,000 pounds of rice. That was all, nothing else; no equipment, no building, no staff; however, these two reasons for my reluctance paled before a third, and personal, concern, the plight of my family, left behind in Beijing. If I went to Chengdu, the distance between us would increase even further. Still there was nothing to do but try to do my best for the bombing victims, and so in May 1939 I left Guiyang for Chengdu.

In Chengdu I found that no progress in health matters had been made during my sojourn of eighteen years outside the province. The missionary schools and hospitals had influenced the health status of the people to some extent, but their work was largely philanthropic and the Chinese themselves had made no serious attempt to promote public health.

I began to organize medical relief for the hundreds of wounded immediately on my arrival. There was no government hospital in Chengdu at the time. Therefore, my approach was to enlist the collaboration of the missionary hospitals and the medical schools of the West China Union University, which at that time was an amalgamated institution embracing the faculties of several other universities that had had to close down because of the war. The university had been established in the early 1900s by Protestant missionaries from Canada; hence, its original faculty was predominantly foreign. In 1939 many Chinese were also enrolled at the University, including one group from Chilu University in Shandong Province, another group from National Central University in Nanjing, and a few former students at St. John's College in Shanghai. The amalgamated institution was quite willing to cooperate in a program to assist the wounded.

Medical relief work occupied me more or less full time until early 1941, when I was able to give some attention to organizing a six-month field training program for rural health instruction of medical and nursing students. With the help of the medical schools of the amalgamated university group, we developed a health service in Wenjiang, a town and district of the same name, near Chengdu, as the teaching facility. A former PUMC student, Li Ting-an, took charge of the program.

After the United States declared war against Japan, an American airbase was established at Chengdu, and antiaircraft equipment was brought in. In time, as resistance against the Japanese stiffened, the bombing attacks became less frequent and finally stopped. We were then able to begin to turn our attention primarily from medical relief to the establishment of a provincewide network of health services.

Developing Urban and Rural Health Services

Meanwhile, I had been appointed Professor of Public Health at the the medical school of the West China Union University as well as commissioner of health for Sichuan Province, a huge and populous province that extended some 700 miles from north to south and some 500 miles east to west. At the time of my appointment there was no public health organization of any kind in the province. Even the city of Chengdu, the provincial capital, had no health department.

A framework of public health service had already evolved in

connection with our medical relief work, however. The temporary hospitals for the wounded; the isolation hospital; various maternal and child care clinics; and a training center for nurses, midwives, and public health personnel, as well as the rural teaching facility had all been organized. In addition, there were antiepidemic mobile medical corps.

We next began to develop municipal health services in Chengdu and district-run health services in the rural districts. By the time I resigned at the close of the Sino-Japanese War, there were more than eighty health centers in the majority of the districts of Sichuan Province. Well-trained technicians and professionals to staff these units were relatively scarce, of course, but essentially the demand was met. Sources of trained personnel included recent graduates of provincial medical colleges and the medical schools of West China University, as well as some older physicians who had come to Sichuan to escape the fighting but who stayed on permanently at the conclusion of hostilities.

With such a large number of rural health centers in Sichuan operated under district government auspices, I felt that during my tenure as commissioner of health, we had made a significant start in the inauguration of state medicine on a provincewide basis. No other province at the time had anywhere near as many rural health centers as had Sichuan.

In addition, total public expenditures for health had increased many times over between 1939 and 1946. Most of the increase reflected expenditures at the local level by district authorities eager to have a health facility in their own jurisdiction for the first time. The provincial budget increased as well, however—exponentially, in fact. In part, the increase was real, indicative of the secretary-general's growing confidence in our program. In part, however, it was attributable to spiraling inflation, which was already terrible, and in the postwar years would reach devastating proportions. From the original Y3,000 our annual operating budget had increased to more than Y10 million.

From this experience in wartime Chengdu, I gained some valuable insights. I saw that it was possible to make substantial progress in developing rural health care delivery, even with very limited economic resources and under very trying conditions, provided the support of government officials and medical college administrators could be enlisted. Also, I acquired additional experience in medical education, teaching quite a number of medical and nursing students who later worked in the provincial municipal and district health organizations. That experience reinforced my belief in the crucial role of practical field training for public health personnel.

The support we had received from the provincial government in Sichuan throughout this period was attributable in part to two related personal experiences. First, the provincial governor had become ill. He registered a high fever, and his personal physician had begun treatment with sulfa drugs. The fever of the stricken official decreased, but he then developed conjunctivitis in both eyes. At that time, I was called in for an opinion and, after examining him, attributed his optic condition to sensitivity to sulfa. My advice was to discontinue use of the drugs. Twenty four hours later the conjunctivitis had subsided markedly. The governor and his family concluded that I was a "better" physician than the highly respected person who treated him regularly.

Next, the mother-in-law of the governor developed lobar pneumonia. The same respected physician initially treated her—successfully, at first, but subsequently she developed an arrhythmic heartbeat. Again I was called in as a consultant and found that her physician had used digitalis, which can cause arrhythmia. Treatment with digitalis was discontinued, and her heartbeat soon returned to normal.

These incidents are recounted as evidence, not of my personal skills as a physician, but underlining that sound clinical training is as important for a public health physician as for any other. In this case, the individual patient benefited from not only my clinical consultations but also the public at large, since shortly thereafter the governor approved a substantial increase in the budget of the provincial health commission, which I headed at the time.

Establishing a National-Level Medical College

After the cessation of hostilities in 1945, that same governor joined the Nationalist central government when it moved eastward from Chongqing back to Nanjing. For the time being, I retained my teaching and administrative posts in Chengdu. In 1946, however, I moved to Chongqing, where I had been asked to establish a medical school at National Chongqing University. Once the medical college became operational, I served as its dean and as professor of public health until 1952. The new institution would be effectively the first regular government medical school in a province of 70 million people.

I had to start from scratch, just as I had done in 1939 in organizing the first provincial health administration in Sichuan. Before taking up my new responsibilities, I made a brief trip to the United States. The Japanese had closed down the PUMC in 1942, and now it was to be reopened. I had been asked to serve on its Board of Trustees, and made the trip in that capacity. In the United States, I took the opportunity to visit Harvard, Cornell, and Western Reserve Universities to examine the public health education programs they were setting up in the postwar era.

Returning to China in early 1947, I went to Chongqing and immediately began to establish the preclinical departments of what was to be the Medical College of National Chongqing University, using a rented building for classroom space. At the same time I was appointed superintendent of two teaching hospitals.

The most immediate and urgent problem was inflation. The allotment with which we had undertaken to establish the medical college had been very small to start, but runaway inflation soon decreased its true value further. Many colleagues thought it would be impossible to organize the college because one could not find faculty even for the preclinical departments who would be willing to work for the small salaries we would offer. In a situation of rampant inflation, everyone was quite understandably concerned about nurturing their economic resources, and clinicians could earn far more in private practice than we could pay.

The solution I decided on was to hire promising young medical school graduates, whose immediate earning potential was less than that of older colleagues, and to give them, in place of a high salary, responsibilities and opportunities for professional growth they could not obtain elsewhere. One of these opportunities was the possibility of a fellowship for advanced training abroad, funded by the American Bureau for Medical Aid to China, a privately sponsored group involved in postwar reconstruction, in whose leadership J. Heng Liu, former Minister of Health, played a prominent role. Through this program, for example, we sent a pathologist, a bacteriologist, and several physiologists to universities in the United States for advanced training.

I selected these prospective faculty members with utmost care, and in time was able to gather a highly qualified faculty, composed of enthusiastic and innovative young clinicians. Only two held the rank of full professor, however, one in biology and the other in pathology. With this faculty assembled, we organized a full six-year medical curriculum, including a one-year internship.

Spiraling inflation, however, continued to threaten the fledgling institution throughout the remainder of Nationalist rule. At one point the equivalent of my entire annual salary was needed to feed my family for just one week, which indicates the severity of the situation. Everywhere people were fighting for food, as the price of rice skyrocketed, not so much because there was a real shortage as because merchants with ties to the Guomindang had stockpiled it to create artificial scarcities. Warlords and landlords in Sichuan Province in particular were making life hard for the peasants, who were preoccupied with a day-to-day struggle for survival. Villages were being emptied as the farmers and their families succumbed to nutritional edema. In the cities, salaried people felt the impact, in particular, and were driven to selling furniture and other family heirlooms to prevent starvation.

Somehow, though, despite the destructive consequences of inflation, the medical college was able to survive and prosper during this difficult period, when the country's resources had been depleted to almost nothing after decades of war, disillusionment, and corruption. We managed by judicious hiring of personnel; by economy in the use of equipment, some of which we shared with other university departments; and by other careful administrative decisions. We had even begun to develop a rural field training site in the Beipei area, about two hours distant from the campus; however, this program had to be discontinued with the escalation of Communist efforts to oust the discredited regime. Aside from having to abandon our field training program, however, we felt we had made credible headway in the 1946–1949 period, overcoming not only the financial problems but also the many academic and other difficulties that inevitably arise in the course of such an undertaking.

Late in 1949 the struggle to liberate the country had reached a climax, and tension among the local inhabitants in Chongqing was running especially high. Corruption and the accompanying political and economic chaos had taken their toll on the city's inhabitants, and rampant inflation had sent morale plunging within the teaching profession.

In November the Guomindang troops based at the Chongqing airfield had fled. Some workers at the medical school and the affiliated teaching hospitals, too, were on the verge of flight. The situation climaxed on the 29th of that month with the triumphant entrance of the People's Liberation Army (PLA) into the city that had once been the wartime capital of the Nationalist government.

PART II

Postliberation China

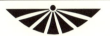

5

The Health Experience From 1949 to 1976

$\blacktriangleleft\!\!\!\ll\!\!\!\blacktriangleright$

Liberation in 1949 found me at National Chongqing University, in Chongqing, serving as dean and professor of public health at its Medical College, which I had organized and established in 1946. That moment in history was one of great optimism in our country, as the Chinese Communist Party (CCP) prepared to assume leadership of the newly established People's Republic of China, proclaimed by Party Chairman Mao Zedong in Beijing in October of that year.

The fundamental commitment of the CCP to the well-being of the common people provided the basis for a vision of a strong, new China, shared by members of the party, intellectuals such as myself, and other segments of the population. Rid of the Nationalist regime, which had sapped the country of its human and material resources, we could at last realistically once again cherish the hope of building a new society. Inflation, hoarding, and speculation, we expected, would soon also disappear, and efforts could be waged to counter the poverty, ignorance, and disease that had so long beset most of the population. As a physician with strong patriotic feelings, I looked forward to contributing to health improvement in the new socialist society.

Like other medical scientists, however, I was not able to contribute much to health development between liberation in 1949 and the death of the party chairman in 1976 and the subsequent overthrow of the radical Gang of Four. In the aftermath of party moves that silenced intellectuals and discouraged their initiative after 1957, it became impossible for me to pursue my personal interest in enlarging the arena of scientific medical activity in rural China. Less than ten years later, the Cultural Revolution in 1966, with its tumultuous impact on the national life, especially in the scientific and academic spheres, still further circumscribed my activities.

In those years, party policy toward intellectuals as a group underwent a series of tortuous ups and downs, and to a large extent my own fortunes mirrored those shifting positions. Still, I fared better than some others. Political authorities permitted me to perform medical relief in the rural areas from time to time. In addition, I was fortunate to be able to continue teaching public health or directing research at a key medical college throughout a part of that period.

Meanwhile, China had advanced toward party goals on many fronts. Overall, progress in health care delivery had been very great. Between 1958 and the late 1960s, the party had succeeded in coordinating the establishment of a rural health care system that extended throughout the country. Given the numbers of people covered, the distances that separated them, and the dearth of resources—both human and monetary—the building of so extensive a system in so rapid a time was an impressive achievement. That feat, in turn, permitted significant strides in the control of epidemic diseases through massive immunizations of the farmers.

The rapidity with which this was accomplished, nonetheless, precipitated uncertainty among some experienced physicians about the quality of patient care, especially at the village level. The great majority of new recruits had had little or no formal education. Thus they entered the system typically lacking a sound grasp of human physiology and of the scientific basis of disease prevention and treatment. Their medical training was brief and unsystematic, not likely to fill in many of these gaps. There seem to have been no definite standards applied, and training varied considerably from place to place and individual to individual. Close supervision of the work of the new recruits could have alleviated some of these problems, but the system had not yet evolved to that point.

In a number of cases the training of even fully credentialed physicians educated in the 1949–1976 period was less than optimal, if only because it had been cut short in midstream. Over much of the period, intellectuals had lost favor, and "expertise" was disdained. Medical studies were shortened and simplified. Often the teachers who taught these abbreviated programs were products of these curtailed programs themselves.

Another feature of the health experience of the 1949–1976 period that had an enduring impact on health in China was the adaptation of Soviet patterns in scientific organization and research, in line with a foreign policy that called for "leaning to one side" in the global struggle between the superpowers.[1] The consequences were particularly significant for public health as a discipline, diverting it from the mainstream of general medicine. From the mid-1950s, public health no longer embraced a broad field of population-based issues but was confined to a narrow set of technical research topics, with emphasis on laboratory experimentation.

Overall, the 1949–1976 period had brought evident progress in health in some respects, while in others the results were less clear. Future years would provide plenty of time for reflection and stocktaking. One issue that seemed likely to be raised at some later date was whether, in the rush to expand the rural health infrastructure after 1958, considerations of quality had been kept in balance with those of quantity.

POSTLIBERATION CHINA: 1949 TO 1976

The well-known political campaigns of this period had major social and economic repercussions, including direct and indirect consequences for health development. The first of these was the so-called antirightist movement that followed on the Hundred Flowers Campaign in 1956/57. In the Hundred Flowers interlude, intellectual leaders in many fields, including medicine, had been encouraged to speak openly and to evaluate progress and programs under CCP rule. Initial response had been cautious, but the invitation in due time produced a wave of comment and suggestion that the party chairman must have found decidedly unwelcome for shortly thereafter the CCP launched an antirightist movement, vilifying those who expressed opposition to party policies and effectively discouraging any further rendering of critical views. Scientifically trained physicians and even some traditional scholar-physicians were included in the group that was rendered mute by the antirightist movement. With those persons silenced, medicine and public health thereafter were largely deprived of the influence of technically trained leadership.

The party launched the "Great Leap Forward" in 1958, emphasizing mobilization for acccelerated economic growth, under an ideological banner featuring themes of national self-sufficiency and labor-intensive production. In the countryside the agricultural cooperatives were organized into still larger socialized collective units—the communes. The communes had both economic and government functions, and their administrative committees were accountable to authorities at the county level. Members of communes were subdivided into brigades and work teams. Farmers were encouraged to have large families as a means of increasing agricultural production.

After several years, the Great Leap Forward was discontinued. Official communiqués blamed its shortcomings on three years of natural calamities, including severe droughts in some areas, and the requirement to repay a large debt to the Soviet Union. An interlude of relative political quiet ensued, during which the views of a relatively more moderate group within the leadership evidently prevailed and the position of intellectuals somewhat improved.

The interlude was short-lived, however, and was followed by the outbreak of the Cultural Revolution in 1966. Much has been written of the chaos and suffering of that period, surely the most traumatic episode in the history of postliberation China, and it is not necessary to reexamine those events in this account, except in relation to its impact on public health and medical education. Chinese and foreign spokespersons alike have commented that the episode represented a "decade of disaster." With respect to science and technologically advanced education, its negative effects were especially felt; medical science had been no less affected than other fields.

HEALTH DEVELOPMENT BEFORE 1958

Immediately after liberation in 1949 the CCP made clear that its approach to health care would contrast markedly with that of the Guomindang. In accordance with socialist ideology, health protection for the entire population would be a central pillar in the new China. Whereas the Nationalist Ministry of Health had been quite powerless, given as a sop to a loyal party supporter and largely ignored by the inside leadership, CCP members immediately below the top-ranking echelon stepped in to run the new Ministry of Health themselves. Its authority was immense, and it began early to plan for a centralized health program under state control.

In 1950 the health director for Southwest China Regional Administration summoned me to his office for a face-to-face discussion of health plans. He indicated that he expected soon to institute a health program in our region, under which everyone would have access to free medical care. I was interested to see how that would be accomplished.

That same year, the government held a National Conference on Health in Beijing, which physicians and other health leaders from across the country, including myself, were invited to attend. Premier Zhou Enlai delivered a six-hour speech containing many allusions to the CCP commitment to work for the people and urging the medical profession to devote itself to serving the country. Four slogans greeted the conferees and suggested the future direction of health policy: "Prevention first; serve workers, farmers, and soldiers; combine traditional and Western medicine; mobilize the masses."

Overall, there seemed to be reason for optimism. The health director for our part of China was endorsing state medicine, and at the national level, officials were talking "prevention first." It seemed as if public health teaching would receive strong support and that attention would be given to control of infectious diseases. Regarding the call for combining traditional and Western medicine, although the party chairman had clearly put his power and prestige on the line in support of the concept, what that might portend precisely we could only speculate. Like most of his comrades, he had spent much of his life in rural areas, where traditional medicine was the common form of medical relief and probably had a considerable amount of confidence in its efficacy. Still, he had also had some experiences that disposed him favorably to scientific medicine. One of the modern physicians attached to the PLA in the preliberation period—missionary-trained Fu Lianzhang, for example, had treated the party chairman successfully for malaria. Fu Lianzhang was later assigned to a high-ranking post in the Ministry of Health. The PLA as a group, in fact, had been generally impressed with the surgical skills of the modern physicians who served with them.

As it turned out, initially the party treated the two systems of medicine rather equitably. As the health bureacracy filled with cadres of rural origin, creating a natural constituency for indigenous medicine, however, there soon were signs that it would receive special attention.

In time, deliberate steps were taken to promote traditional medicine by broadening knowledge of it among modern physicians and by increasing the number of formally educated practitioners. Short courses in traditional medicine were introduced into the modern medical curriculum, and new colleges of traditional medicine were established in many cities. Terminology adapted from modern medicine began to infiltrate the lexicon, possibly to give it added legitimacy for scientifically oriented persons.

Party support for traditional medicine was troubling to a few modern physicians at that time. For anyone wrestling with the health problems prevailing in rural areas of our country in the 1950s, however, it was a pragmatic and not unrealistic policy. The rural population did not have access to any other form of relief, and to undermine its confidence in the traditional system under those circumstances would have been an irresponsible action.

Many of the new functionaries of the Ministry of Health had at one time been PLA medical workers. Some of them had received instruction in surgery or other areas essential to keeping an army healthy and on the move. By and large, however, their opportunities for formal education had been few and far between; what they knew came mainly from experience gained in the field.

Underpinning operations in the new health administration were two important working principles: (1) scientific work could, and should, be centrally controlled; and (2) in the framework for control, scientists themselves would be responsible to government and party functionaries who would make the policy decisions. Those functionaries, of course, were, in turn, responsible to the high-ranking officials in their own institutions for program development and execution. Many physicians—chiefly those with modern training, but also including a few scholar-physicians—failed to understand this new arrangement of working within a bureaucratic framework under administrators with little or no formal medical training.

In this context the reconstituted Chinese Medical Association, of which I served as vice president from 1951 to 1956, naturally exercised little voice in health affairs. It conducted business as usual for a few years, experienced a short-lived merger with an association of scholar-physicians, and then was placed under the direction of the Ministry of Health. Members of the board, formerly appointed, were henceforth chosen by the ministry. Once subsumed under the ministry, however, the CMA had little influence, functioning mainly to support the execution of policies formulated by administrators.

Even at the start of Communist rule, when the CMA had had some autonomy, it exerted only a minimal influence on general medicine and public health. The only subject that seemed to arouse much interest within the CMA, or from those responsible for its activities on the outside, was surgery. This held particularly true when it came to representing our country at international conferences, most of which were held in Soviet and eastern European bloc countries. Typically, it was surgeons who were sent to publicize medical advances in the new China to the outside world. It was not without irony that many of surgeons representing China had been trained at the PUMC, which in the light of its former foreign connections was being subjected to voluminous criticism by Chinese authorities at the time.

Strengthening its ties to other socialist countries, and seeking to learn from them, China was heavily engaged in remodeling its medical education and research organizations. Health and medical resources were being funneled into the construction and development of large urban hospitals, teaching institutions, and research organizations. Many high-ranking officials were sent abroad on study tours, while lower-ranking functionaries were brought together at locations in China.

I, myself, was sent to the Northeastern Provinces to study Russian models in public health training. Having taught myself the Russian language, I was asked to translate a public health text for use in the secondary medical schools that were operated by provincial government authorities.

In the early 1950s, China critically lacked physicians. Qualified medical school instructors were even more scarce. Accordingly, under a new policy in effect with the academic year 1952/53, the medical school studies program was reduced from six to four years for the sake of rapid turnout. As a solution to the shortage of faculty, a number of relatively inexperienced young instructors were recruited and given short, supplementary medical courses intended to compensate for the deficiencies in their backgrounds. Older professors had trouble adapting their instruction to the new simplified program, which bypassed much of the clinical material and laboratory experimentation of an earlier period.

The policy was modified after only one year amid fears about the quality of future health care expressed by the general public as well as by physicians. Another year was added to the medical curriculum, bringing the total to five. This arrangement remained in effect until 1958.

Medical school programs addressed the needs of students preparing for clinical work in urban or county hospitals or research institutions, and attention to the public health content of the curriculum soon became quite perfunctory. The general topics covered in public health studies—all superficially—were vital statistics, environmental sanitation, industrial hygiene, child health, nutrition and food hygiene, and pest control. The approach was based on the work of Max Joseph von Pettenkofer, a nineteenth-century German professor of medical chemistry. Content focused on such matters as the physical and chemical properties of air, water, soil, and food, with little attempt to relate these to social or biological conditions. The textbooks tended to duplicate materials covered in preclinical and clinical courses, especially material dealing with infectious diseases. Epidemiological case studies were notably lacking. Classroom instruction occupied over 50 percent of the time. Field training diminished to the vanishing point, and graduates emerged with no real sense of broad public health issues. Not surprisingly, medical student interest in public health diminished radically.

Meanwhile an experiment in medical education had been launched in the Northeastern Provinces to train a group of physicians specifically for practice in rural areas, where 80 percent of China's nearly one billion people live. Under the program junior-high-school graduates were enrolled and given a three-year program of medical training. The program was subsequently extended to other parts of the country. Graduates were variously known as "physicians" or "physician's assistants."

Meanwhile, medicine and public health education began to go

separate ways. The Minister of Health had shown an interest in such an arrangement as early as 1950, and in 1953 the ministry organized a pilot program of specialized public health training. In 1955 the matter was formally concluded, with the announcement of plans to discontinue training of public health physicians and to organize instead separate public health schools for the training of "public health specialists."

Each of the six key medical colleges was to have such a school. One of the six was Sichuan Medical College, which had been organized on the campus of the former missionary-operated West China Union University, and when its public health school was established, I became its acting dean.

Officials of the Ministries of Health and Education formulated the overall framework of a generally four-year curriculum for the new public health schools. It was to cover two to three years of preclinical and clinical instruction, without much practical work, and less than one year for different public health specialties. As the program evolved, it emphasized classroom and laboratory instruction rather than field training at rural sites, where problems existed and required solutions. Graduates of those schools, rather than physicians, were to be the vanguard of new public health leadership.

The new schools accepted high-school graduates for training from the same pool of candidates also being considered for medical, dental, and pharmaceutical training. Although the public health schools were on the same academic level as the schools of medicine, they ranked lower in prestige because the best students were selected for medicine, not public health. Not unexpectedly, science and clinical teachers were quite uninterested in the public health students. Teachers in the public health schools were nearly all trained on short courses of different specialties without practical experience.

THE GREAT LEAP FORWARD AND THE
LAUNCHING OF A RURAL HEALTH
SYSTEM

In the years that coincided with the Great Leap Forward, there was a surging interest within the CCP in mobilizing the farmers in support of CCP goals and, in this context, in providing support to meet their special needs, including health. Intellectuals and others who were neither farmers, workers, nor soldiers were held in low esteem, and educational attainment was generally devalued. Consistent with this political view emanating from the top, medical education was shortened once again to three years after 1958 in most schools. (A few remained under the five-year arrangement.)

High-level interest in the needs of the agricultural population was absolutely crucial to the massive expansion of rural health care system that took place beginning in 1958. Without it, this achievement would certainly have never been accomplished so rapidly and perhaps might never have occurred at all. With it, all the power of the central government, and the leverage that power provided, was brought to bear on the task. Given the impetus of the authority and prestige of the party chairman, the buildup proceeded with a degree of speed and deliberation that could hardly have been imagined in the past. In fact, there was so much centralized power that the government could achieve almost anything it set out to do.

While central and provincial health officials had voiced both the desire and the intent to extend modern health care across the country, until the highest authorities intervened, the idea had largely failed to materialize. They had built a few small hospitals in some county seats. Apart from that, however, efforts to date had concentrated on the operation or construction of hospitals and clinics in urban areas in a pattern not unlike the one that I had observed in the Soviet Union some years before.

The agencies that operated these facilities included, besides the Ministry of Health, the health administrations of the provinces and a number of other province-level government organizations, including three municipalities. All were urban-based bureaucracies. They formed the upper-level and urban component of government, as distinct from lower-level and rural component—the counties, subcounties or communes, and villages or brigades.

Health officials were called to task soon after the Great Leap Forward began. The Ministry of Health came under sharp attack, as Chairman Mao criticized its urban orientation and charged it with being "the ministry of influential people," serving only high officials.

The initial response to the criticism was to dispatch mobile health teams to provide some clinical care to the farmers. Mobile units could go only where roads took them, however, and so proved to be of limited use. More importantly, the mobile clinic teams were stunned by the magnitude of need they encountered in rural market towns and villages, especially by the incidence of infectious disease. The authorities thus began to plan some measures of prevention, albeit somewhat hesitantly, as the ideas of some officials about preventive medicine were rather vague.

Before prevention programs could be carried out, however, the rural health system had to evolve. This was to be accomplished through rural administrative organizations and depended on full-scale cooperation from county authorities and input from sub-county and commune representatives. County hospitals were already in evidence and county health bureaus were organized or upscaled at this time; however, the most significant development of this period was the development of organizations at the commune level. Ninety percent of communes developed a health facility of some type.

Initially these typically offered either traditional or modern medical care, but not both, and were supported in a variety of ways. The first were cooperative clinics with a traditional practitioner in charge, whose upkeep depended on patient fees. Later subcounty officials and commune committees opened a number of small hospitals and health centers staffed by salaried graduates of secondary medical schools. In time, all three types of facility were combined into commune health centers, in which the patient could obtain either modern or traditional care. Besides providing a relatively large amount of health service, the commune centers trained some village-level health workers in elementary medical work.

EXPANSION FROM COMMUNE TO
VILLAGE: THE 1960s

The significant strides made in the control of infectious disease through massive immunization were made possible by the huge aggregate of village-level personnel assembled mainly from 1960 onward. The main component of this aggregate consisted of "barefoot doctors," who, for better or for worse, served as prototypes for many other developing countries as they organized their own rural health services. The barefoot doctors were not, however, the only persons giving immunizations and doing primary health care in Chinese villages in the 1949–1976 period. In immunization work, midwifery, and later, family planning, lay people contributed substantially.

The rural health system that had evolved by the mid-1960s was three-tiered, consisting of the county health bureau at its apex, with commune and village-level facilities below that. The county hospitals had come first, mainly before 1958; the commune health centers next, between 1958 and 1964; and the village clinics at different times between 1960 and 1970 or so. Apparently there was a great deal of overlapping in the development of health organizations below the county level, and the whole picture became rather confusing. About all that can be said is that the system developed from the top down, and whatever facilities opened in the communes and villages resulted from decisions of higher authorities.

It is almost impossible to clearly differentiate between the time when village health workers, with little training, and the time when barefoot doctors, with considerably more training, were turned out. About all we know is that barefoot doctors first entered the picture in the early 1960s, and that their number increased greatly during the Cultural Revolution. Some were traditional practitioners or lay health workers who had entered the system as affiliates of commune organizations. Others had been doing practice of traditional medicine or selling herbs in their own villages before becoming barefoot doctors. County hospitals trained some of them, a few for periods of from six months to a year. Commune and subcounty organizations trained others.

The practical training of these barefoot doctors varied from case to case, of course, although presumably the common ground consisted of instruction in a few simple medical procedures and in techniques of immunization. The time came, nonetheless, when many barefoot doctors were doing considerably more than that, with some doing diagnosis and treatment on the same level as ordinary physicians. Given the variation in their backgrounds and abilities, not to mention those of the persons who trained them, their caliber varied widely. Some were considerably less proficient than others.

Even the most competent, however, had to practice without any planned support from scientific and technical personnel with more advanced training. For there was no suggestion of developing a carefully structured system, such as we had organized at Dingxian, which linked such workers to a hierarchy of more fully trained medical personnel at higher rural levels, or to advanced scientific personnel in the cities. To the contrary, their responsibilities were ill defined, and, lacking systematic supervision, they were free to act most of the time entirely on their own judgment. On a quantitative basis much was achieved in the massive rural health expansion, but later there were indications that the quality of village-level medical care would have to be considerably improved through programs of further training in a post-Mao system.

During the Cultural Revolution universities established branches or teaching points in rural areas. This gave further impetus to rural health development and the system, establishing firm roots in the villages. Also, young teachers were diverted from classroom duty and sent as permanent residents or members of mobile teams to serve the rural areas and to assume some of the responsibility for training additional barefoot doctors. Health directives issued from the top were channeled through new provincial health administrators who replaced the more experienced personnel.

The push to train barefoot doctors ended about 1972, and perhaps one-third of the total group returned to full-time farming, when funding for the activities became problematical. Rural health continued to develop, although at low standards.

HEALTH POLICY AND ITS IMPACT: A MID-1970s PERSPECTIVE

MEDICAL AND PUBLIC HEALTH EDUCATION

Meanwhile in the 1960s, medical education in the universities had gone through another cycle of extension and attrition. In 1963 the three-year curriculum established in 1958 was adjusted upward to a full six-year curriculum. The Cultural Revolution, however, led to a reversion to the three-year curriculum once again in 1968, as supporters of the CPP party chairman assented to the idea that even primary school graduates could become medical doctors. In

1972 there was a final upward readjustment once again, echoing popular disillusionment with the Cultural Revolution policies.

The impact of all this on the modern medical field can be assessed when we consider that between 1949 and 1978 almost two generations of medical professionals were produced, while the older generation, trained in accordance with the preliberation six-year curriculum, was moving into retirement age. It was difficult to remain convinced that faculty and students alike, including those students who became teachers after graduation, had not been placed at a disadvantage by these shifting arrangements. Whatever the case, the end result very clearly was great variation in the scope and substance of medical training. Diversity became so great, in fact, that what a physician, physician's assistant, or barefoot doctor trained in this period had or had not studied was an unknown variable.

As for public health education, the pattern of early specialization had continued throughout the period. Theoretically, early specialization had strengthened the discipline. In reality, year after year, premature specialization produced graduates who were ill-prepared, especially because of their lack of clinical training and scientific background. To some teachers, too, they appeared to have failed to gain an adequate understanding of the broader meaning of public health. Students were unable to supplement their deficiencies through self-study. In the final analysis they were perceived as health professionals of little use. Perhaps as many as 40 to 50 percent became discouraged and entered other careers. Public health education then became an enigma to those of us who had received a different type of fundamental training.

THE ALTERNATIVE SYSTEMS OF MEDICINE

By the mid-1970s, the gains for traditional medicine could be seen in both rural and urban areas. In the countryside, traditional medical practitioners were working together in the same clinics with modern-trained secondary medical school graduates. In the cities, where Mao's ideas had permeated hospitals, clinics, and medical schools, comparable developments had taken place. There were, of course, separate traditional medical hospitals, but in some modern hospitals specific areas had been designated in the outpatient departments for traditional medical consultations. Varying numbers of traditional and modern physicians thus often worked side by side under the same roof, although the patients for each type of practice were kept separate. Each system had its own pharmacy, too, but modern physicians were being encouraged to learn how to prescribe traditional drugs.

Separate departments of traditional medicine to be found in the national and provincial health ministries had been authorized to develop traditional medicine on a wide basis. Plans included the organization of special hospitals of traditional medicine in each province and county. Such plans were readily received by the people, who believed in the usefulness of traditional medicine, especially for the treatment of chronic disease.

A MEDICAL SCIENTIST IN THE NEW
SOCIETY

As to my personal participation in the Chinese health experience during these years, it had been largely in the capacity of medical educator. Nonetheless, I had also had some opportunity to engage in rural health work in outlying parts of Sichuan Province, and in Yunnan Province, a neighboring province to the south. Initially also I had participated periodically in various conferences and study sessions in other parts of the country.

By the time of liberation in 1949, I had been living in Chongqing for three years and was deeply involved in getting the new medical college at the national university on its feet. This presented endless problems. A fairly strong faculty of medical science was built up in spite of the disastrous inflation. With two teaching hospitals of over 300 beds, the six-year curriculum was carried to completion for the first class of medical students, who graduated in 1952. The CCP meanwhile had accumulated an excellent record in halting the spiraling inflation of the preliberation period.

Graduation of the first class in 1952 provided a moment of personal fulfillment and patriotic pride to many of those involved. In the past most of our medical graduates had come from missionary-run teaching institutions and after completion of their studies had been drawn into the network of modern hospitals and clinics in the cities. Now, however, we had a national university medical college in our own province that we had built entirely with our own resources, and whose graduates were well prepared to work for the benefit of the common people in a newly liberated China. Many would be recruited to work in the provincial health administration or would become professors in different medical specialities.

In 1952 I took eighty students to Yunnan Province on the border of Burma for field training (see fig. 2 inset). There we studied malignant malaria and bubonic plague among the minority nationality people at Mangshi, a large market town some distance southwest of Kunming. A surgeon and an obstetrician accompanied us on the trip, which took twenty days by truck, a portion of it by way of the historic Burma Road. Villagers in the area relied on traditional practitioners exclusively, except for a few more affluent peasants who crossed the border into Burma, where they paid a very high price for modern medical attention. Thai people predominated among the three minority nationalities in that sector of Yunnan Province. The area was then under military control by the PLA, but an old tribal government headed by a Tusu chieftain survived.

Mangshi had a small clinic, with a few beds. We rearranged the limited space into consultation rooms and an operating area. Suspicious at first because they had been badly treated by Chinese in the past, the people came around after a few months of hard work on our part, treating patients with terminal and other conditions and performing preventive work. They began calling on us in a variety of situations.

As a field experience for the students, it was a rewarding interlude, giving substantial insight into health problems among the rural poor and how the application of scientific medical knowledge might elicit improvement. A number of students subsequently became leaders in health organizations serving rural populations.

We reduced the incidence of malaria after mass drug treatment and educated people to use mosquito nets and to open their windows to permit sunlight and ventilation in their houses. We performed surgery, attended cases of difficult childbirth, and treated cardiac failure, all with some success. The people had the habit of depositing their feces around the villages, to be eaten by the pigs. Since they also ate meat raw, a very high percentage of the population was infested with tapeworms. When patients were treated and saw the worms they had been harboring, they were greatly surprised. We then gave some simple lessons about contamination.

We returned home in March 1953 to find that the CCP had taken over all administrative positions, including the deanship of medical schools. For me, this meant that I would be relieved of administrative responsibility but would continue to teach. With the absorption of the Medical College of National Chongqing University by the Sichuan Medical College, my family and I moved to Chengdu, and I quite comfortably started to undertake only public health teaching to medical students. My lectures were well received by the students, and I was to begin my field instruction. The new government was already emphasizing classroom and laboratory instruction, however, so it became necessary to teach epidemiology without field studies.

In Manchuria, where I had been sent in 1950 to study new patterns in medical education, I had already seen evidence of trends that seemed to me to somewhat jeopardize the quality of medical education. The stress on classroom lectures, using poorly translated Russian texts, the use of a provisional three-year curriculum, and the passive attitude of students during clinical demonstrations that I had seen all were disappointing. Also disconcerting was the interest in early specialization for public health students evidenced in Beijing at the First National Conference on Health. The neglect of field training was another milestone for me in a journey in the wrong direction.

Then in 1955, I was sent to Beijing to attend the conference of medical educators, at which it was made known that separate public health schools were to be established. A number of persons at the conference were unable to understand the principles underlying the announced curriculum. Participants, however, were not expected to discuss the decision. Whatever our views, a colleague from Shanghai and I were both appointed deans of new schools of public health.

Having made a number of criticisms of the general trends in medical education during the Hundred Flowers Campaign, I was later removed from the deanship and downgraded from second- to fourth-grade professor, with a loss of salary and certain amenities. Thereafter my teaching conformed strictly to official method-

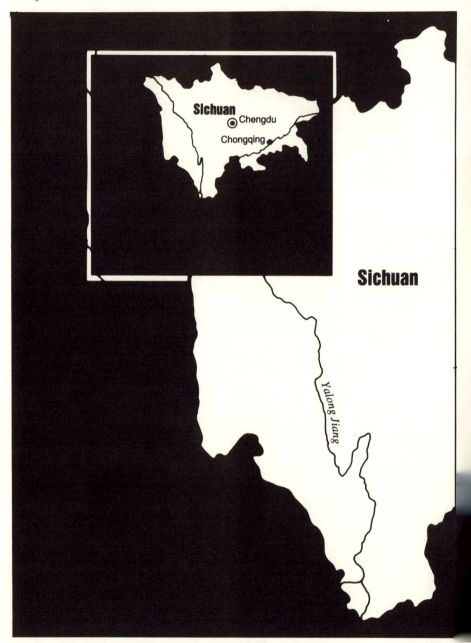

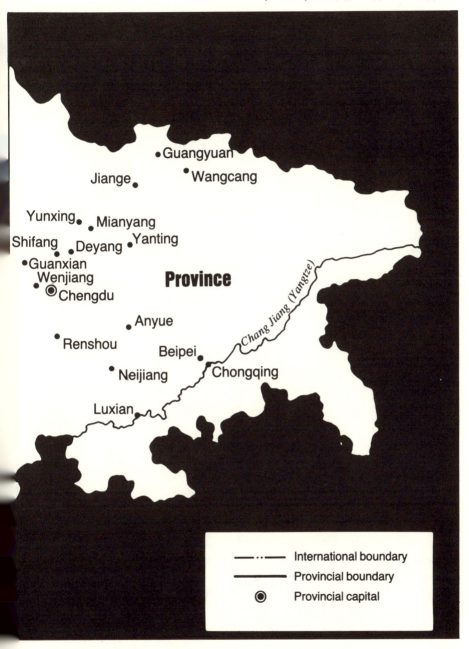

Fig. 2. Observation and fieldwork sites, Southwest China, 1952–1986.

ology, and my contact with students was more or less restricted to formalities.

Intellectuals had been criticized for preferring the cities and not being willing to help the common people, so between 1958 and 1966 I was twice sent to rural areas to render medical relief. From my own perspective, this was a welcome assignment, for it gave me an opportunity to observe rural conditions firsthand and, as I was still a teacher, to utilize the situation to provide some students with field training. They responded quite well, and we had a good time together.

The 1958 assignment was to provide medical relief in a northern area of Sichuan Province where leprosy and syphilis were prevalent. Travel from Chengdu to the destination in the northwestern corner of Jiange County took one day by train. I was accompanied by other teachers from the Medical College and a number of students.

In the principal population center in the county, there was a thirty-bed hospital with an army medical officer in charge. The officer spent his time in the hospital and had no firsthand knowledge of health conditions or problems in the surrounding area. As expected, the local inhabitants depended almost entirely on traditional practitioners for such medical care as they could obtain.

What we saw and experienced in Jiange County made me realize once more just how scientifically unenlightened villagers were and the extent to which superstition and fear still permeated their ideas about disease and its cure. For example, although traditional practitioners had an abundance of theories, neither they nor the army medical officer seemed to have any practical knowledge of diagnostic procedures. So one day I invited a group of eighty or so for a brief talk on the subject. To illustrate the talk, I brought in a few typical patients with leprosy and syphilis into the classroom. Confronted with the patient with leprosy, the traditional practitioners became greatly alarmed. Their anxiety was so great, in fact, that when I examined the patient in their presence, many covered their eyes and buried their heads, evidently fearing that they might contract the disease simply by looking at a diseased victim.

That field trip also made me realize how essential it is for anyone in public health to have a good foundation in scientific medicine, both curative and preventive. One day on a visit to Wangcang and Guangyuan Counties nearby to the east, we saw an increasing number of leprosy cases. In one small village, I was introduced to a man who for years had believed he had contracted leprosy. After careful examination, I found that what he actually had was psoriasis, not leprosy. On being informed of this, the man jumped for joy, shouting that he had received his second life. Had the original diagnostician been more knowledgeable, that patient might have been spared years of suffering. No doubt, concurrently, there were many actual cases of leprosy going undiagnosed and untreated. This reinforced my conviction that it is essential for rural public health workers to be thoroughly familiar with diseases prevalent in the areas in which they work.

By 1960 my status had begun to improve, and gradually restrictions on my activity were relaxed. In time, I was permitted to travel to certain areas, read certain materials, and participate in a number of conferences, all of which had previously been prohibited to me. In 1963, for example, a conference was held in Beijing in an attempt to raise the social standing of the intellectuals and to make for a more comfortable atmosphere, downplaying some of the criticism that "rightists" had received. I was treated as a guest for a few days.

In 1964 several colleagues and I visited rural areas in Anyue and Neijiang Counties, southeast of Chengdu. The Neijiang Regional Health Center was responsible for preventive work in the area, a subject of much interest to us. Disappointed, we found that it was spending most of its resources on laboratory examinations of water and food. Its epidemiological surveys were confined largely to areas in the immediate environs of the city. In the city of Anyue the water supply was quite inadequate, and surface pollution of drinking wells was evident everywhere.

Later I reflected on the importance of systematic organization in rural health care delivery and concluded that intermittent visits by mobile health teams simply cannot do the job. Without systematic organization, the tendency is toward hit-or-miss measures of prevention, while attention is concentrated on institution-based health activities in the urban pattern. Physicians think in terms of the needs of patients in hospitals and clinics, while those of the community as a whole are often neglected.

Another field trip in the same year took me to the Yongxin commune, in Mianyang County, north of Chengdu. A commune health center had not yet been established at that time, but there were clinics in three market towns, two practicing modern medicine under the direction of a secondary medical school graduate and the other run by traditional practitioners. One of the modern clinics specialized exclusively in schistosomiasis, and we established ourselves there. Although our diagnostic capabilities were considerably better than those of the young secondary medical school graduates, without any laboratory work, our findings were inconclusive.

After working there for some time, it became quite evident that the quality of health service in the clinics of the area was low. The personnel assigned to antischistosomiasis work engaged in some snail eradication. But neither they nor the clinic personnel had had sufficient training for what they were expected to do.

The poverty prevailing in some villages compounded other problems. This was brought home to us by the case of a woman we encountered in a field. Obviously ill, she was greatly in need of some drugs for which we were expected to charge a negligible fee, but she could not afford even that small sum. Fortunately, a friend helped her out. That incident convinced me that economic improvement of impoverished areas is always a necessary corollary of lasting health improvement.

At Sichuan Medical College, the impact of the outbreak of the Cultural Revolution on academic life was immediate. Intellectuals once again immediately became targets of criticism. In 1966 new admissions were suspended. In 1968 they were resumed but this time only for a limited number of junior- and senior-high-school graduates who came on the basis of official recommendation rather than on the basis of a competitive entrance examination as in the past. The institution was moved to the rural areas and classes were conducted mostly by young teachers of peasant or worker origin. Students were given short courses in which political considerations took priority over medical content.

In 1972 classes were reinstituted on the Chengdu campus. Professors and other staff members were called back to work. On my return, the party asked me to do only technical work. Given a choice of several alternatives, I finally decided to study the diagnosis and treatment of occupational lung diseases that attacked many farmers working in the mines. This decision was approved by the party.

Between 1972 and 1975 I became the first scientific leader of research on occupational lung diseases. By the end of 1975 my vision became very poor and I tendered my resignation. This was accepted, and I left the college to retire in Beijing. I was in that city when the Gang of Four was overthrown in 1976, paving the way for the emergence of a new national leadership.

6

A New Era in Health Development

In 1978 postliberation China entered another phase in its history, and with it my own life passed another turning point. A rightward shift of the political pendulum not long after the death of Party Chairman Mao in 1976 was reflected in the rise to power of a pragmatic reform group, headed by Vice Chairman Deng Xiaoping. In its emphasis on expediency, the reform group adopted a strategy of concerted mobilization for development, launching a campaign of economic modernization whose ambitious targets, if realized, would propel China into the ranks of relatively advanced, industrialized nations by the year 2000. The drive to make modernization a reality has continued unabated over the past decade, carrying socialist China in new directions under strong party leadership.

With science perceived as the key to modernization, advanced scientific and technological training was valued once again, and intellectuals collectively were now treated with respect that had been unknown for decades. After the Cultural Revolution was declared at an end, intellectuals all across the country began returning to their posts. I myself was asked to come out of retirement, and returned, at the request of Sichuan Medical College, to my former position as Director of its Occupational Lung Disease Laboratory.

In the drive to make modernization a reality, policymaking and administrative arrangements assumed utmost importance. With so much concentration of authority in the central government, and in some cases in the provincial government, the formulation of correct policies and their execution through appropriate and effective administrative channels was absolutely critical to the future of the modernization movement. This was true of all constructive efforts, including health improvement.

Somewhat surprisingly, emphasis on modernization had not carried over into medical practice to any significant degree, although science and technology represented one of the "four modernizations" (modernizations in agriculture, industry, science and technology, and defense). Instead, in the decade since emphasis on modernization had begun, traditional medicine had further reinforced its institutional position and in the late 1980s stood on an equal footing with scientific medicine.

Trends in modern medical education were nonetheless consistent with the country's need to build and maintain a scientifically skilled medical community. The institutional structure of higher education in modern medicine had been strengthened, and the general course requirements that had prevailed between 1963 and 1968 had been reinstated. By 1987, a five-year curriculum of advanced study had been standard in most medical colleges for a decade, while a few leading educational institutions offered programs of six or more years.

The same time period passed, however, without reexamination of the patterns of public health education that had been imposed under Soviet influence more than twenty years earlier. Public health education in 1987 therefore continued to be based on the assumption that its work was better left to "specialists" who are not medical doctors and whose training followed a rather narrow channel of interest, rather than to physicians trained in public health. In medical school itself, public health studies are deemed significantly less important than clinical coursework. Because some public health "specialists" become disappointed with their choice and change to other careers while others disappear into large bureaucratic institutions in the cities, public health in rural areas depends largely on the younger, less experienced graduates.

It was, nevertheless, impressive to see the great amount of work that has actually been, and was being, done to improve health in the rural areas, through antiepidemic campaigns, health services for women and children, and other means. In many places the upward turn of the financial situation of farmers under economic modernization had resulted in better living standards and had been accompanied by increased demand for medical and health care. In other areas where, in late 1987, financial conditions were not so good, village household budgets did not permit discretionary spending for health protection or improvement.

With respect to health improvement in the villages, perhaps the most difficult challenge facing the new leadership was the high percentage of untrained physicians and other medical workers serving in rural China—a legacy of efforts at rapid extension in an earlier era. Even those physicians who had received some formal instruction had been disadvantaged by disruptions and dislocations in medical education in the same era. Seemingly, the only solution for this troubling situation was the provision of systematic training programs for health personnel of all types by local authorities.

POSTLIBERATION CHINA: 1976 to 1987

Chairman Mao died in September 1976; his wife, Jiang Qing, and her three associates were arrested in October and subsequently exiled. China had been in a chaotic state at that time, and the question of succession that arose in the aftermath of Mao's death was not settled for several years. By 1978, however, the issue had quite clearly been resolved in favor of Deng Xiaoping and moderate elements within the party, who by that time had risen to occupy many of the key leadership positions in the party and the government.

The pragmatic reform group confronted an array of problems, not the least of which was that, thirty years after liberation, the country had little to show in the way of economic growth. Moreover, its population had increased from 540 million to roughly one billion. This made China the world's most populous nation, creating enormous demand for food, housing, jobs, education, and health care.

The strategy of response involved economic modernization in four areas: agriculture, industry, science and technology, and defense. An emphasis on orderly and pragmatic processes of change, to which intellectuals were expected to contribute as a group, replaced the revolutionary shifts of the previous period and the belief that scientific and technical work could be done by persons without specialized training. Ambitious plans for what were termed the "four modernizations" were widely publicized through mass campaigns to nurture patriotic feeling and encourage youthful enthusiasm.

In time, scientists were afforded some freedom of initiative in research that contributed directly to modernization. A widely heralded national conference of sciences was convened in Beijing in March 1978, and in the same year Deng Xiaoping declared intellectuals to be members of the working class, after which they were regarded as equal in social status to workers and peasants. The scientific and intellectual community was encouraged to participate in a two-way exchange of information with their counterparts in technologically advanced countries, the flow facilitated by a new "open-door" policy in foreign affairs.

While official interest not unexpectedly focused on the physical sciences, within limits social sciences were strengthened as well. Before 1978, Marxism was considered the only legitimate social science discipline, but in 1979 in the more open-minded environment a Chinese Academy of Social Sciences was established with responsibilities for promoting scientific studies of social phenomena on the basis of worldwide knowledge. Soon afterward, Sichuan Province established its own such academy.

Decisions reached by the Central Committee of the Party in December 1978 set the stage for a series of economic and political reforms whose full realization would produce fundamental change in many aspects of the national life. The implementation of general reform guidelines, however, starting in urban China, commenced at a modest pace, as reform-minded innovators made small headway in persuading old-style administrators to adapt new habits of thinking.[1] From 1984, however, after many old Party retainers in provincial and county administrations had been replaced by younger reform-minded functionaries, we began to see some change.

TRENDS IN HEALTH POLICY AND ADMINISTRATION

In health administration, the pattern was more or less the same. Specifically, in the early 1980s a few leading physicians in central research organizations and major industrial territories began to express opinions, take the initiative, and try to influence persons in positions of authority. Technical service organizations and the medical universities received a few benefits from these initiatives. Meanwhile the minister of health had been removed from office and was succeeded by his vice minister.

In general, however, administrators at the provincial level and below were slow to implement reform guidelines as they might apply to medicine and public health. To a number of the older bureaucrats, many of whom were former army medical workers, the suddenness of the ideological turnabout was quite incomprehensible, and they found themselves perhaps unwilling, or perhaps unable, to follow through. Younger men and women appointed as county health bureau directors or superintendents of county hospitals during 1984 and after were more reform-minded.

In 1982, with encouragement from the World Health Organization, the Ministry of Health targeted several county health systems to serve as models and began to look for professional input into these systems. I was approached for advice on rural health personnel and their training.

The changed political climate made possible the convening of a national conference of community medicine in Chengdu in 1984. Most of the delegates at the conference were young, technically trained supporters of the new leadership. Many papers were presented dealing with health conditions in the rural areas. One result was the organization of a National Center of Public Health Administration at Sichuan Medical College. My experience in developing rural health services was again recognized, and I began to advise its staff on field training activities.

POLICY RELATED TO TRADITIONAL MEDICINE

Within the central health administration, the creation of a new Bureau of Traditional Medicine in 1984 seemed to signal encouragement to practitioners and supporters of the style of medicine venerated in China over so many centuries. The proliferation of new hospitals, clinics, and schools of traditional medicine seen in the early to mid-1980s reinforced this impression. What the benefits and costs of the policy placing the two systems of medicine on an equal footing might be for future generations remained to be seen; for the present, however, most Chinese seem to want to go along with the equitable treatment.

Accordingly, in just about every area of medical education and practice, agencies and facilities representing both traditional and modern systems may be found. Each system has its own representation in the central government, as well as its own nationally or provincially administered urban clinics, hospitals, and medical schools. At the county level, there are typically also traditional as well as modern medical hospitals, although the major share of funding seems to go to the modern facilities.

As of 1987, organizational conflict has almost entirely disappeared. In the cities modern physicians and scholar-physicians treat patients in some of the same hospitals, and in the countryside secondary medical school graduates and traditional practitioners work side by side, without constraint, treating patients according to their own individual principles without thought of criticism from the other practitioners.

Freedom of choice for the patient can produce interesting results. This was impressed on me in 1979, for example, during a field trip to Deyang County in Sichuan Province. There I visited what was then called a *commune health center*, where traditional medicine was practiced. It was very busy, full of patients. A dozen "doctors" were prescribing drugs. A few streets away there was a government-run modern health facility. The contrast between the two was startling. The modern facility had only a few patients and its staff had very little to do.

The situation aroused my curiosity. What could explain it? Wherever the two medicines (of which neither is standardized) were available, they were undoubtedly rendering some useful service. So why was the preference so strong? Perhaps only because of long ingrained habit. Perhaps, as I was inclined to think, however, it could be explained in part by shortcomings in the training of modern physicians serving the farmers, which diminished popular confidence in them and made them appear less competent as a group than traditional medical practitioners. Whatever the reason, more training for modern physicians serving in rural areas would be to the advantage of our country.

POLICIES RELATING TO VILLAGE HEALTH

In the years between 1978 and 1987, a number of economic and social policies had strong effects on the life of the farmers. Apart from the dramatic increase in prosperity in some areas resulting from modernization reforms, perhaps the most obvious was the reduction in births proceeding from the strictly enforced policy of one child per family.

In 1987, in the counties whose circumstances I am familiar with, contraception is widely practiced, as in other rural areas, although some farmers still want more than one child. Barrier methods, sterilization, and abortion for both married and unmarried women are the most common methods; barrier methods have a 20 percent failure rate, however, and numbers of women become pregnant unintentionally. Chemical preparations are not very well favored. For the married, all surgical operations and treatments of possible complications are free of charge. For the unmarried, there is a charge, assigned in accordance with government regulations.

The benefits of family planning for improved child health are readily evident. With smaller families, household financial circumstances have been upgraded and living conditions improved. All but a very few parents are prepared to spend money to guard their child's health, and they are careful to do so.

The situation reinforces the assertion I had made nearly forty years ago in Chongqing to Dr. Marshall Balfour of the Rockefeller Foundation: public health without birth control may do more harm than good for Chinese farmers. I am now 100 percent in favor of our family planning policy, notwithstanding certain side effects, to whose long-term consequences—both social and emotional—our government is highly sensitive. The government, in fact, has already taken steps to ameliorate such affects.

In one of the model counties of Sichuan Province, Shifang County, which I visited in 1986, now almost all young parents have only one child, and with only one, they take painstaking care of the child's health. Parents pay close attention to immunization, knowing its importance, and reports indicate that 88 percent of the children have been immunized under current control programs. Some parents, on discovering that their child was not given a vaccine when others were, will not rest until they are satisfied that the child was already protected.

Other directives, including several issued in 1985 by the Ministry of Health, also had important overall and long-term implications. One of these created a new category of physician, the "country doctor," ranking intermediate to the regular medical school graduate and the "barefoot doctor." The "barefoot doctor" who can claim to have passed a formal examination is entitled to the new rank.

Most of those who became country doctors through this new regulation are, in fact, traditional practitioners with a modest overlay of scientific training. The likely inference, then, is that traditional medicine will gain an additional advocacy group, one with more influence and prestige than barefoot doctors or village health workers, and that scientific medicine may be set back farther.

The creation of another category of "doctor" added to an already confusing situation. The term "doctor" had come to have only a very loose meaning. Persons with academic degrees in modern medicine, graduates of secondary medical schools, traditional practitioners, barefoot doctors, and now country doctors, as well as persons who simply prescribed and sold drugs, were all referred to as "doctors." No criteria have as yet been established to distinguish among these various and, to some extent, overlapping categories, notwithstanding the great variation in their qualifications to practice medicine.

Two other regulations were of interest in terms of their potential for affecting health in rural China, one permitting "barefoot doctors" to engage in private practice, setting their own fees, and the other permitting private entrepreneurs to manufacture and sell drugs for profit. Because "barefoot doctors" in general have had less than optimal training, and because China suffers from a scarcity of published medical reference material, many rural physicians lack a sound understanding of the scientific principles on which the use of certain drugs is based. As private practitioners, however, they are legally entitled to prescribe drugs without restriction, under little or no supervision. This can put the patient at considerable risk.

Also, the temptation to pursue monetary profit may be irresistible for a few barefoot doctors. This would be difficult for the farmers, who depend on them in health matters and respect their judgment. Rural inhabitants already tell visitors of alleged incidents in which a barefoot doctor has prescribed an injection for only slight illness or has substituted inferior medications for a more costly one.

The private production and sale of medications also had troublesome implications. Until 1985, rural physicians could obtain drugs only at government dispensaries, These dispensaries had been the exclusive agents of all drugs, of which the government was the sole manufacturer. Now, however, physicians may not only prescribe drugs without supervision but also purchase them from any supplier they choose, and any individual who elects to produce drugs may do so. In theory, the quality of drugs purchased from all sources is the same. Private drug manufacturers are subject to official monitoring of standards by a quality-control bureau. The proliferation of small companies makes it increasingly difficult to exercise full control, however, posing the danger that the quality of privately produced pharmaceuticals will fall significantly below that of those manufactured by the government. The current government is still the main drug producer, but its share of the market seems to be declining.

Party and government leaders are not unmindful that problems could develop and in 1986 clearly indicated their commitment to the well-being of farmers and strengthened movement for positive change in their behalf. In that year alone, the Ministry of Health sponsored two major meetings at which delegates focused on rural health concerns and local training issues. Both meetings took place in July of that year in Shandong Province, one a national conference of medical educators held in Qingdao, the other a national rural health conference held in Yantai. Out of the latter movement came the movement to organize a permanent consultative body, the National Rural Health Association. These were highly significant developments and, all in all, it would be difficult to understate the importance they held for discussion and long-term constructive action for rural health.

Meanwhile other forward steps were also being instituted by the national leadership, some with input from international development agencies working in China since the implementation of the open-door policy. The agencies included the United Nations Children's Fund (UNICEF), the World Health Organization (WHO), and the International Bank for Reconstruction and Development (more commonly known as the "World Bank").

Such agencies had an important influence on health policy and administration, although their contribution was usually indirect. For example, when Ministry of Health officials shifted from generally impromptu discussion as a basis for planning and evaluation to scientific methods employing quantitative analysis, foreign technical personnel were consulted for advice as to the best methods for setting up a new statistical bureau in the ministry.

In another example, there is, in our own province, the Shifang model county health program. The World Bank lent support in its establishment and continues to provide some technical assistance; but China runs the project. Shifang County government functionaries and health officials are responsible, and some respected medical and health figures serve as special consultants. I personally, as a professor of community medicine at Sichuan Medical College (now renamed West China University of Medical Sciences), offer suggestions on health training and other matters.

ORGANIZATION OF HEALTH SERVICES

The organization of health services in China today can be described in only broad terms. The system exhibits regional and local diversity and is subject to organizational rearrangements at any given time or place. Even terminology shows no obligation to hold still.

About all that can be said with certainty is that the Ministry of Health, in the central government, is the source of, and final authority on, planning, policy, and budget matters, and all other health agencies are ultimately accountable to it. The Minister of Health is a member of the State Council, or Cabinet.

In the implementation of policy, the Ministry of Health provides technical supervision through a chain of agencies linked together down to the lowest level, the village (see fig. 3) All health agencies, both urban and rural, generally implement central government decisions without modification, although a recent ruling, taking account of the country's great diversity, allows a few provincial governments somewhat more freedom than others. Units at each level

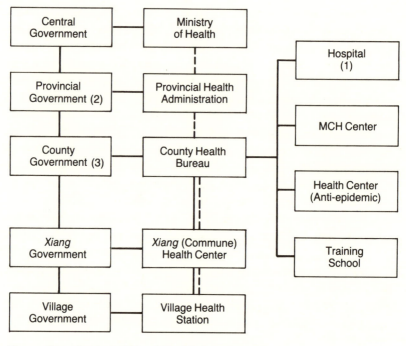

Fig. 3. Organization of Rural Health Services, 1987

1. Some counties have a traditional hospital as well as a modern hospital.

2. In some provinces, there is a regional level of administration between the provincial and county levels, with its own regional health center.

3. In some counties, there is a subcounty level of administration between the county and the *xiang* levels, with their own subcounty health centers.

———————— Administrative authority, including policy, budget and personnel.

– – – – – Technical supervision of programs.

select their own staffs, but appointments are subject to approval at the next higher level.

Below the Ministry of Health there are more than twenty province-level governments, including municipalities and autonomous territories, having their own health administrations. Some province-level units are divided into regions having their own health administrations.

All these agencies as well as the hospitals, schools, and clinics they operate are government facilities, staffed by government employees. Together they constitute the urban component of the health system, as distinguished from the rural component. The distinction between the two components is significant and has many implications for sources of funding, personnel, and other matters.

The rural component of the health system dovetails with the urban component at the county level of government. County-level governments (the apex of authority in rural China), and the county health bureaus they operate, enjoy considerable autonomy in selecting personnel and carrying out day-to-day operations. They are, nonetheless, ultimately responsible to provincial health administrators, who, in turn, are accountable to the officials of the Ministry of Health.

The organization of health services below the county level varies from place to place. In general terms, however, it can be considered as a three-tiered arrangement consisting of units at the county, *xiang*, and village levels. (The *xiang* administration replaces the disbanded communes.) Each of the three administrative tiers has its own responsibilities and functions and operates different facilities. While this arrangement resembles the three-tiered organization at Dingxian in 1930, which encompassed district, subdistrict, and village-level units (and it does entail arrangements for technical supervision), it seems to lack the emphasis on integrated functioning that we considered to be the essence of the Dingxian system.

The general scheme was modified in certain counties, however. Some counties actually have a four-tiered system with an intermediate subcounty level between the county and the xiang level.

The staffs of county-level agencies throughout China are salaried government employees and, like others in that category, are entitled to free health care. In North China—the generally poorer half of the country's traditional heartland, government employment in health generally extends down to the xiang level of health administration, meaning that the staffs of local health facilities at that level have access to free medical care, as do urban government and factory employees. This is seldom the case in South China. Rural health everywhere, however, is supported in various ways, particularly including the provision of subsidies for preventive work.

As to health agencies below the county level, they, too, receive some subsidies, mainly for equipment. By and large, however, the local community provides resources for their establishment and operation; treatment costs are borne by individual patients.

THE URBAN COMPONENT

The Ministry of Health has general responsibility for the health and well-being of the population, although family planning matters are essentially the responsibility of another ministry, with which the Ministry of Health only cooperates. Additionally, the ministry operates various educational, research, and treatment facilities in Beijing and some other cities. These include what are called the "key medical colleges," as well as a number of hospitals, and scientific research institutes.

Among others, the research institutions include the monumental Chinese Academy of Medical Sciences (CAMS), with a total working staff of more than 10,000 persons, which was formed by merger with the PUMC and another medical institution.[2] The CAMS has yielded a number of high-level research projects against important epidemic diseases, including plague, schistosomiasis, kala azar, and venereal disease. One recent CAMS research project led to a breakthrough in treatment of uterine cancer.

Intent on improving academic standards in higher education, the post-Mao leadership restored the competitive entrance examinations for all prospective university-level students and lengthened the medical school curriculum in regular and key medical colleges to six years or more. In another policy decision, it established departments of community medicine in a number of medical schools.

Quite a few representatives of these new departments attended the National Conference of Community Medicine held in 1984 at Chengdu. Since then a professional journal has been established, and some university departments have launched plans to conduct regular classes for the training of health administrators. As of 1987, however, the scope of activities of the new departments was not yet well defined.

Province-level health administrations also played a key role in urban health care and medical education. A great many of the hospitals and clinics in Chinese cities are administered by provincial and municipal governments, some constructed in the pre-1958 period when much attention was devoted to development of urban facilities and others more recently in the drive for modernization. Some hospitals engage exclusively in scientific medical practice, others practice traditional medicine exclusively, and still others have sections or facilities for either.

Not unexpectedly, while these facilities are all located in the cities, their patients are not exclusively urban. The reputations of the provincial hospitals reach out to the countryside, and in serious cases those villagers who are discontent with the rural medical care and who can afford to come to the city to seek help will often do so. For example, in early 1986, I encountered a well-to-do farmer whose broken fibula had been improperly handled at a xiang health center. When he obtained no relief from treatment by local physicians, he sought help from a highly respected orthopedist at the provincial hospital.

This influx of farmers to urban hospitals is a trend worth noting. Provincial hospitals are already heavily burdened with urban patients, and the influx of villagers imposes an extra load on provincial hospital staff physicians. Because of this patient overload, the staff is hard pressed, and some may be left unsatisfied with their treatment. Moreover, the trips are costly for the farmers who often must wait for several days before being admitted to the hospital and must find, and probably pay for, temporary lodgings somewhere.

Key medical colleges, located in major cities and operated by the central government, are the most prestigious medical schools devoted to teacher-training responsibilities. Usually, schools of dentistry, pharmacy, and public health are affiliated with each medical college. A traditional medical college in Beijing, administered by the central Ministry of Health, is among the key medical schools.

Provincial authorities operate the other two types of modern medical college—the regular medical colleges and the lower-rated secondary medical schools (which accept junior-high-school graduates for admission), plus some schools of traditional medicine. As of 1987 there were about 100 provincial medical colleges and about 500 secondary medical schools.

Test scores on the basis of general competitive examinations determine the order in which students can select the medical, dental, pharmaceutical, or public health school of their choice. Because the public health field is not well understood, public health schools are seldom selected first. About one-eighth of the successful medical college candidates are assigned to traditional medical colleges, which under the present administration enjoy almost the same professional standing as modern medical schools. The four-year curriculum in these schools generally consists of an initial two years of scientific study, including courses in pathology and biochemistry, followed by two years of traditional learning.

As to course requirements in public health schools, there is considerable emphasis on laboratory work, entailing examination of air, water, food, and waste products, or animal experimentation. Field training, through which students might profitably be exposed to major health problems in their country and possible solutions, is greatly downplayed. Many graduates are absorbed into provincially administered health research institutions, where examination of various aspects of epidemic, endemic, and occupational disease is conducted. Others join the county-operated anti-epidemic stations.

Ranking below the key and provincial medical colleges are the secondary medical schools, which train junior-high-school graduates for service as physicians in rural areas. On the basis of the number of years they had been in operation, and the average class size, by 1987 these schools presumably graduated nearly one million physicians. The schools also train some nurses and a few midwives for rural service.

Clinical training in the secondary medical schools is quite brief; thus, graduates cannot be assumed to be anywhere near as skilled as regular medical college graduates, who in the rural system are concentrated at the county level. Their reputation as a group seems to be declining. They are at an apparent disadvantage even compared with many "country doctors" or "barefoot doctors," who may have had little formal training but who have benefited by their considerable practical experience. A 1986 survey reports that among those country doctors evaluated, 75 percent were rated as equally competent or more competent than a physician who had graduated from secondary medical school.

The issue of competency and the need for field training and local training school activity for the benefit of many health personnel was made further evident by statistics published in the mid-1980s by several provincial governments. For its part, for example, the Sichuan provincial government recognizes four grades of "doctor" and two of "medical assistant." Of "doctors" enumerated in the province in 1984, 13.7 percent were college-grade, meaning that they had graduated from a regular or key medical college; 24.8 percent were junior-college-grade, meaning that, on the basis of their experience, they were deemed more qualified than the secondary medical school graduates at the next-lower level; 38.5 percent were secondary-medical-school-grade; and 23 percent had had no formal training whatsoever. Among the medical assistants, 64.28 percent were secondary-medical-school-grade. The remainder, almost one third, had had no formal training of any type.

Zhejiang Province has the highest educational levels in China, but even there many of the "doctors" were totally without formal medical training in 1984. According to official figures for that year, only 19 percent of physicians in the province had graduated from a regular or key medical college; 46 percent had graduated from a secondary medical school. But again more than 33 percent had had no formal medical education.

Meanwhile a survey in the same year from Heilongjiang Province provided further indication of just how critical was the need for additional systematic training. In a sample survey, asked to comment on the proficiency of a group of 100 physicians, respondents categorized 22.7 percent as "competent," 51.9 percent as "not competent," and 25.3 percent as "very incompetent."

Because the better-trained and, therefore, presumably more competent physicians prefer to work at the county level and above, such distributions fall particularly hard on the farmers. More than likely, the least qualified physicians are to be found mostly in rural areas.

THE RURAL COMPONENT

The general scheme of rural health services has evolved over the past thirty years. What I know of that system, of course, is based on my familiarity with the situation in my own province and does not necessarily pertain to, or characterize, circumstances in other parts of China.

The County Bureau of Health

The function of the County Bureau of Health is to execute policy designed by higher authorities and approved by local party officials. In this context it engages in both curative and preventive work. Funding comes mainly from the county budget, with small additional increments from the provincial government. The range of total health expenditures probably varies considerably from one county to another and from one part of the country to another. Precise information on this point is not available.

The county health bureau serves as administrative headquarters and provides the most technically advanced level of services available. The service agencies in counties in our province, and in many other Chinese counties, include one or more hospitals (some counties have both a traditional and a modern hospital and sometimes a specialized hospital), a health center, a maternal and child health center, and a training school for continuing health education.

The county hospitals are the apex of the medical care service agencies. They have the most advanced equipment and the most specialized staffs and are supposed to attend to the most seriously ill patients. While physicians trained in secondary medical schools still constitute the majority of staff members, an increasing number of graduates of regular medical colleges are now being appointed to serve with county hospitals.

A county hospital that has the best equipment, specialized manpower, and a dedicated staff may still face many resource deficiencies and technical problems; thus, even the finest county hospital might be unlikely to qualify as a model for rural medical care. The staffs are short-handed. More nurses are needed to relieve families of patient care responsibilities, more nutritionists are needed to attend to special diets, and more architects and engineers specializing in hospital design are needed to focus on such special aspects as water supply and waste disposal. Because many medical personnel have little knowledge of the nature of infection, cleanliness of the surroundings is not a high priority. Even physicians and nurses may fail to assign high priority to cleanliness; for instance, it is by no means unusual to hear that the surgical incision of a hospital patient became infected because the site was not kept unscrupulously clean.

Regardless of what the term "county health center" implies, these facilities generally are intended not for dispensing treatment but for preventive medicine after the Soviet model. Their main responsibilities are communicable disease control, health services in schools and factories, public health education, food hygiene, and collection of vital statistics. Some counties also operate special health centers for endemic disease, such as filariasis.

The maternal and child health centers offer various advisory and oversight services. For example, they provide health care and information on nutrition to pregnant women. After a child is born, they offer regular health examinations, monitor growth, and plan immunizations.

The training schools for health offer continuing education courses for local health personnel. Teachers are drawn from the staff of the county hospital.

Xiang-Level Health Facilities

With county hospitals caring largely for only the most seriously ill patients, the real burden of providing medical relief for a rural population of some 800 million persons falls to the xiang and village-level facilities and personnel. Of the former, there were, in 1981 (according to a report circulated at an international health conference in Singapore in 1981), some 554,000 health centers, averaging fifteen beds each, with a total staff of 935,000. Since then, some consolidation had taken place, with the more accessible and best equipped xiang health centers being upgraded to form so-called key centers, with oversight responsibility for about five smaller health stations in the surrounding areas. Statistics for 1987 are unavailable.

When commune health centers were first organized in the late 1950s, they were financially supported in different ways, ranging from a majority that were completely, or very largely, supported by the commune to a minority organized on some sort of a fee-collecting basis. In recent years, the government has advocated a change-over to a fee-for-service arrangement for all xiang health centers. Xiang-level health authorities are accountable to county officials, but in planning and supervising village-level personnel whom they are responsible for supervising, they have some degree of autonomy.

Xiang health centers provide a wide variety of patient care, treating serious cases of infectious disease and surgical need as well cases of minor illness or injury. They also are concerned with preventive activities, provision of health care for women and children, and family planning. Typically the staffs included one or more secondary medical school graduates, but in many cases personnel had received only on-the-job training.

Performance of surgery by persons lacking sufficient training is, of course, strictly forbidden. Nevertheless, this seems to occur occasionally when, for one reason or another, physicians overestimate their own capabilities. A rumor circulating in a rural county in 1986, for example, concerned a farmer who experienced bleeding for two weeks following an ineptly performed vasectomy. The farmer was unable to work while recuperating and lost his entire income during that period. Circulation of such stories or rumors could have an adverse affect on the entire birth planning program.

Village Health Stations

The days in prerevolutionary China—when, for example, 220 out of 472 villages in the rural district of Dingxian had no medical facilities of any kind—are gone forever. According to the latest data available to me (from the 1981 conference held in Singapore), China in 1981 had 670,000 village-level health stations, covering 85 percent of all villages. Affiliated with them were 1,348,000 barefoot doctors, 30 percent of whom were women. Additional affiliates included 1.6 million village health workers and about 0.5 million midwives.

Such stations are usually staffed by two or three people, but this number may vary depending on the size of the village. The county government subsidizes the station for its family planning activities and immunization projects. The village provides the treatment rooms and some equipment and medicine. The affiliated barefoot doctors charge fees to the patients for all services including immunizations, which until recently were given free.

The functional distinction between the barefoot doctors and the health workers is somewhat blurred. In general, however, at least in Sichuan Province, the former concentrate more on curative medicine and the latter, on preventive measures. The health workers, who work only part time, earn small fees and engage, for example, in malaria control or health propaganda activities.

Immunization programs were suspended in some places during the Cultural Revolution, except for smallpox immunization, which was continued by popular demand. Since 1978, however, these programs have been resumed, and the Ministry of Health has assigned them a high priority. Volume and coverage have been widely extended, probably exceeding the level of effort at any time in the past. These immunization campaigns, planned by the authorities and carried out by village-level workers, provide one of the major health success stories of the party (CCP) and the government. Life expectancy in China has risen from 40 years of age in 1949 to 68 in 1986, and infant mortality has declined from 200 per 1,000 live births to 34 per 1,000 in the same period. Rising socioeconomic levels contributed to this achievement, but a major share of the credit is attributable to the immunization campaign programs.

In 1987 immunization activities at the local level remained critically important. Unless immunization were administered by people living in the villages, who could follow those who needed vaccination until the work was completed, the level of infectious disease—regardless of whether the government assigns the issue high priority—could not be controlled. Agricultural work demanded that adult members of farming household be at work in their fields, and they could not accommodate their schedules for those of a visiting mobile health team. Instead, the barefoot doctor with fresh vaccine had to seek them out.

The mobilization of village level workers for preventive work has been accompanied by another trend, however, whose long-term implications are far less laudable: the tendency for barefoot doctors, most of whom are trained only to administer first aid or treat mild cases of common illnesses, gradually to regard themselves as fully trained physicians capable of practicing medicine.

This poses a frequently serious risk to the farmers. In one case, for example, a barefoot doctor treated a patient with acute abdominal pain by injecting morphine. The patient, who actually had acute appendicitis, suffered a visceral rupture and developed peritonitis. Even physicians with many years of medical education are not always skilled at diagnosis, so the dangers of permitting those with only minimal training to do so are obvious.

THE SHIFANG COUNTY HEALTH SERVICE:
A CASE STUDY

It may be useful to share some information and personal impressions gathered in 1984 and 1986 trips to Shifang County, the model county for which I serve as a consultant on rural health training. While general impressions may be valuable, however, China's size and diversity must be constantly borne in mind. Conditions in Shifang are unique to that county and may or may not reflect those in other parts of the country.

Shifang County lies on the northwestern border of the West Sichuan plain, an 863-square-kilometer (850-km²), kidney-shaped area. Eighty percent of its 384,000 inhabitants live in one or another of nineteen scattered xiang. Its northern sector is hilly and mountainous, and its southern sector is a densely populated, fertile plain, watered by the 2,000-year-old Guanxian Irrigation Works. Rice, wheat, corn, tobacco, and a plant yielding edible oil are among its agricultural products. The area under cultivation averages less than one-sixth acre per person, a plot—if carefully cultivated—just large enough to provide food for one person.

Prosperity is evident in many parts of Shifang County today, in striking contrast to the poverty and isolation of twenty, thirty, or forty years ago. Great changes have occurred since liberation in 1949. Agricultural productivity, measured in monetary terms, made a nearly fivefold gain and industrial productivity, a more than fiftyfold gain in the 1949–1982 period. Primary school enrollment rose from 7,000 in 1949 to 56,000 in three decades. Whereas in 1949 there were no hard surface roads at all, today villages are linked to a network of such roads that cross the county.

Like most other counties, Shifang has a health center that serves as an antiepidemic station. It also has a modern hospital with 160 beds, a traditional hospital with 60 beds, and a special hospital for treatment of skin diseases. A maternal and child health center and a country training school for health are also operated in this model county. There are, of course, also the usual outlying xiang health centers and village health stations.

In the early 1980s about Y640,000 was expended for health, the equivalent of about 5 percent of the county's annual budget, and representing Y1.69 per capita. The county hospital received the

largest single allocation, Y140,000, apart from a Y152,000 sum designated to grants in aid to xiang health centers. The antischistosomiasis program, the antiepidemic health center, and the maternal
and child center received smaller sums. Only Y11,000 was allocated
for the county training school for health. Individuals spent an estimated Y6.00 for drugs.

Declining mortality rates and increasing life expectancy provide
telling testimony to recent health improvement. By 1984, according
to official county statistics, the crude death rate was 6.84 per 1,000,
the infant mortality rate was 27.24 per 1,000 live births, and the
natural increase rate was 1.5 percent. Life expectancy was 68.77
years for men and 71.18 for women.[2] These rates compared favorably with those for the more developed countries of the world,
which averaged a crude death rate of 9 per 1,000, an infant mortality rate of 19 per 1,000 live births, and a natural increase rate of 2.0
in the same year.[3]

Cardiovascular disease was the leading cause of death in the
county, responsible for 210.0 deaths per 100,000 persons in 1981. In
the same year, malignancy, cerebral hemorrhage, and accidents
accounted for 63.07, 66.47, and 71.96 deaths per 100,000 persons,
respectively. Other major causes of death were chronic respiratory
disease, gastrointestinal disease, and tuberculosis.[4]

While rising life expectancy and declining mortality were cause
for satisfaction, morbidity data yielded a less positive picture.
County statistical records revealed a high incidence of some infectious diseases even while local surveys indicated that many cases
of infectious illness went unreported. Hepatitis, for example, is
widespread. Tuberculosis is still a serious problem, as is infant
diarrhea and dysentery.

For whatever reason, infectious disease rates in rural areas seem
to be dramatically higher than those in urban areas. According to a
mid-1980s government report, only 2 percent of patients in urban
hospitals run by provincial administrators were being treated for
infectious disease, as compared with 27 percent in county facilities
and 95 percent in xiang-level facilities.[5]

According to a recent estimate, as much as 40 percent of serious
infectious disease cases in Sichuan Province are not reported. Regardless of whether this estimate is high, it might reflect an equally
high incidence of infectious diseases in other parts of China, which

would be of great concern for health authorities. Presumably, the underreporting is attributable to apparent diagnostic failures. Many physicians in rural areas, for example, recognize cases of hepatitis only when they have reached a very advanced stage, by which time family and friends have been exposed to infection.

Observations in 1984

I made several trips to Shifang County during the mid-1980s to observe health conditions. The first was in 1984, on which occasion I visited several xiang health centers and village health stations.

The health center at Luo Xian was relatively prosperous. Operating on a surplus, it was able to utilize its profits for building repair and the purchase of new equipment. Patients paid to register and were charged for whatever drugs were prescribed, at fees set by government regulation.

A staff of thirty-five attended a caseload of approximately 400 patients each day. Although it included only one regular medical college graduate, the center provided care for all but the most seriously ill patients, who were referred to the county hospital. A number of barefoot doctors were associated with the center on a part-time basis, all of whom had received some training at the county hospital—some for as long as two years. Nonetheless, according to a center spokesperson, as a group they would benefit considerably from further training. Lack of qualified personnel and of necessary equipment, in that order, were the two most serious problems at the center, according to the same spokesperson.

The twenty-nine-member staff of the smaller, fifteen-bed Mianzhu health center, made up entirely of barefoot doctors, also trained at the county hospital for periods of up to one year. Common illnesses included bronchopneumonia, bronchitis, skin infections, and hepatitis. Eleven active cases of tuberculosis had just been identified. Poisoning from organic phosphorous fertilizer was not unusual. Many older persons suffered from hypertension. One morning I watched several physicians receiving new patients and making diagnoses. They took pulses but not temperatures and, as far as I could see, undertook no physical examination of chest or abdomen. No laboratory tests were ordered.

Half a mile from the center there was a village health station, served by two barefoot doctors, one practicing traditional medicine exclusively. Colds, entiritis, dysentery, and chronic bronchitis were treated. The physicians collected fees of which they kept a portion, turning the rest over to village authorities.

At another health station, three barefoot doctors served the villagers, two women and one man. One provided medical care, another provided preventive care, and the third was involved with family planning. While the basic responsibilities were distributed in this fashion, all three medical workers had been trained at the xiang health center and knew how to treat accidents, strained muscles, and other common complaints, as well as how to administer injections. Village health workers assisted the staff, preparing so-called common drugs, performing snail eradication according to traditional formulas, and keeping the vital statistics register.

In the same year I was also able to visit the county training school for health in Renshou County, not far from Chengdu. Closed during the Cultural Revolution, the school had reopened in 1980 with a staff of eighteen and facilities for 180 students. Most of the students, I learned, were barefoot doctors or other types of medical aides. While most of them had been rural health workers since the early 1970s, attending this school was the first opportunity they had thus far had to receive any formal preparation for the work they were doing.

Although the training school had three teachers with scientific backgrounds, the other eight were traditional practitioners, and the primary emphasis seemed to be on the teaching of traditional medicine. Anatomy and physiology, for example, were not taught systematically. Elementary coursework spanned general principles of traditional medicine; Chinese drugs; prescription for treatment; and classical theories regarding internal medicine, surgery, and pediatrics. Advanced coursework focused on traditional medical classics. Some clinical work in the local county clinics followed the classroom studies. Students enrolled for anywhere from three months to two years.

Walking around the school, which had four classrooms, I saw only a few teaching aides: some models of human embryos, a few types of pathological specimen, some anatomical drawings, and a few books and journals. One student showed me his textbook, which was one used in secondary medical schools.

Observations in 1986

In April 1986 I returned to Shifang County to observe its primary health care conditions, and the visit provided some interesting comparisons. In the interim, implementation of the new economic policies had infused the farmers and their wives with enthusiasm for creating lucrative activities. Some had banded together to operate small enterprises, such as a cement factory. Other ventures were coal mining, marketing handicrafts, or leasing small tractors for transport. Wives were raising chickens, ducks, and pigs to gain more cash income. Through these endeavors, per capita income had increased from Y350 to Y503, a marked rise in household income. As the number of children had been reduced, discretionary funds were used to add to or build new farm houses or to purchase bicycles, fashionable clothing, or more expensive foods. While a general climate of prosperity prevailed, a healthy young farmer seeking a license to sell ice cream or a group of older men whiling away daytime hours playing cards suggested the existence of pockets of underemployment in parts of the county.

One of the most remarkable consequences of social and economic policy was the reduced size of the family, which, in turn, had resulted in increased care for the sick, particularly the precious one child. It was evident that our success in family planning in the rural areas was making a critical contribution to overall reconstruction. In fact, the lowered maternal mortality rate of 1 per 1,000 live births and the infant mortality of 27.2 per 1,000 live births was directly attributable to the family planning program.

On our visit, we made an on-the-spot investigation of the condition of medicine, antiepidemic activities, health services for women and children, and family planning at the county, xiang, and village levels. We also visited some farmer's homes to learn something about their living standards, culture, and medical and health conditions. Our general impression was that health work was being carried out broadly and deeply. The achievements were highly impressive, and there had been a noticeable improvement in the physical well-being, spirit, and outlook of the local population.

Antiepidemic work was formulated in principle on a nationwide basis by the Ministry of Health, supervised by the county-level health (antiepidemic) center and organized and implemented by xiang and village-level personnel. In Shifang County results were highly impressive, although the funds provided by the county health bureau for these activities were insufficient. Other less serious problems also remained to be solved, but in general the success of the program could be credited with contributing significantly to a decrease in morbidity from infectious disease in the county. Vaccines against measles, epidemic meningitis, tuberculosis, rabies, diphtheria, tetanus, and leptospirosis were in use.

A cold-chain arrangement to ensure adequate refrigeration for vaccines over the distribution network now covers the entire county, donated by UNICEF. That equipment strikes me as the most useful contribution of a foreign agency in the health field, far more so than such equipment as high-power microscopes and rotating slide projectors, which few persons know how to operate.

The public was responding positively to prevention efforts. In 1984, for example, of the target number of cases vaccinated in the county measles immunization campaign, 99.5 percent were actually done; in the BCG campaign 92.7 percent were done; and in the whooping cough and poliomyelitis immunization campaigns 93.6 percent and 97.4 percent, respectively, were achieved.

In each xiang center one or two persons were assigned to work on disease prevention, planning immunizations, and the operation of the cold chain. On the thirteenth day of each month vaccines were sent to the center from the county health (antiepidemic) center. The staff members immediately summoned the barefoot doctors and assigned work to them. A refrigerator was used to store the vaccines, which could be kept for only one week. The barefoot doctors were told to take the vaccines to the village stations and to complete their work by within two days.

After accepting an assignment, the barefoot doctor takes the vaccines in a cold storage packet and goes directly to the village. The women's leader in the village has meanwhile announced the impending immunization program at the school. Parents take the children to the barefoot doctor's home, who may visit from house to house. The cold chain generally seems to be working effectively; however, villagers report that a few barefoot doctors carry the vaccines around with them without too much regard for its safety. This should be discouraged, because when the vaccine is not kept sufficiently cold, the 100 percent acceptance rate becomes meaningless.

Financing the arrangements can be a problem as costs sometimes exceed the sum provided by the county health bureau by 100 percent. In vaccinating children, there is generally no problem in carrying out the work or collecting money to cover the cost, except for those parents who occasionally balk in the winter, fearing that children may catch cold by rolling up their sleeves or removing their clothing. Not infrequently, however, workers encounter resistance from adults, who may be too busy in the fields, or may regard vaccinations as necessary only for children. Some villagers also may be less interested in vaccinations for themselves or their children now that they must pay for something once provided free of charge.

The new regulations on private practice raise further concern that the issue of vaccination will receive less attention, since providing immunizations is not very lucrative for the physician. Most of the Yo.1 fee has to be turned back in to the authorities, with the physician keeping only Yo.03.

Apart from immunization work, considerable success had been achieved in the county in preventing and treating schistosomiasis since an antibilharzia station had been founded. The plan was to eradicate the disease by the end of the year. It was said, too, that malaria would be eradicated the following year. Morbidity from tuberculosis stood at 640 per 100,000 however, and morbidity from hepatitis was also relatively high. Infant diarrhea was a serious concern.

After familiarizing ourselves with the spectrum of disease and efforts to prevent it, we proceeded to study the available medical work in the county, the focal point of which was the well-equipped, well-staffed Shifang County People's Hospital. The equipment of the hospital was adequate and reliable, its staff was of good quality, and a variety of medical specialties were represented. Modern medicine was practiced there, but the county also operated a traditional hospital and a skin disease hospital, which were not included in our visit.

We also visited the training school for health, another county-level organization, which offered a two-year training program. Most of the teachers are staff physicians from the county hospital, soundly grounded in theory and with extensive practical experience. One of several problems confronting school officials, however, is that workloads of the physicians who also serve as teachers are heavy, often preventing them from conducting their classes as scheduled.

At the maternal and child health center we spoke to two secondary medical school graduates who headed the staff. They were supported by other physicians who had studied at the county training school for health and other staff aides. Most of the Y100,000 income that the center earned in 1985 came from fees for pre- and postnatal care, but the county government also provided a subsidy for outreach activities in women's health care.

Theoretically, the xiang health centers took care of patients less critically ill than those sent to the county hospital but more seriously ill than those seen at the village health stations. In part because of decreases in morbidity from infectious disease, some xiang health centers received fewer patients than in the past and, accordingly, were experiencing some financial difficulties. In Shifang County people now have bicycles, and villages even usually have tractors. Thus it has become quite easy in recent years to transport people to the county hospitals.

Whether a given center was in difficulty or not depended on many circumstances, including the location of the center, the convenience of transportation, the numbers of residents in the community, whether they specialized in certain kinds of cases, the skill and reputation of the physicians on the staff, the number of retired staff members, and the relationship between the center and the village government. Only one or two health centers we visited had a regular medical college graduate on the staff.

The tasks of the health centers are more or less the same. They maintain fixed hours and a fixed timetable for work and have four main responsibilities: management of antibilharzia programs, other preventive activities, provision of medical care for women and infants, and family planning. Their laboratories are equipped for routine tests only. For women of childbearing age, the centers are responsible for providing contraceptive information and performing abortions. Unless they are deemed inadequately equipped, they perform first-trimester abortions, but second-trimester patients are sent to the county hospital. The centers also perform sterilization procedures on request. In Shifang County, tubal ligations are becoming a popular method of female sterilization.

A new and recent challenge for those in Shifang has been the decision to provide retirement income for aging staff, reflecting the new retirement policies adopted at the county level since 1984. The difficulty arises from the way this is being done. The retired physician is retained at 75 percent of the former salary, while another person, usually a family member, friend, or acquaintance and not necessarily trained for the work, is added to the staff. For this reason, in some cases retired members may outnumber other members of the staff, imposing a heavy financial strain on the facility, while the new distribution of the workload may increase the burden of some staff members.

Barefoot doctors and country doctors affiliated with xiang health centers and village health stations are doing very well. Typically they continue to farm but do medical practice on the side, serving perhaps twenty or persons in their own locales, or possibly, by dint of good reputation, drawing additional patients from other areas. The typical fee is Yo.7 for a diagnosis and Yo.5 for an injection. They may prescribe either modern drugs or Chinese herbs, for many physicians use both systems of medicine. The patient pays not for the prescription as such but for the cost of the drug, plus a surcharge for the physician of 15 percent on standard drugs and 25 percent on Chinese herbs.

Under current regulations, barefoot doctors in many areas of the country are earning quite a good income. In Shifang County at least Y100, and at most Y200 to Y300 per year, exclusive of income from field harvest and trade sidelines. In the Shanghai metropolitan area, it is reported that those with the best reputations may earn as much as would a professor of internal medicine in a medical college.

While most patients seem to be able to afford the expense of treatment, poorer farmers may seek credit or delay treatment, especially at times when seasonal income fluctuations have temporarily reduced family resources. Another alternative is to ask for treatment in accordance with the resources that are available; for example, the patient may ask for treatment worth Y1. Our impression is that physicians will generally extend credit, although a rare few have been known to refuse.

The quality of physician care in rural areas is contingent on not only the physicians competency but also the utility of medications dispensed. Thus we were interested in visiting the government-run Shifang Medicine and Pharmacy Company. The company conducts a large business, selling about Y2.4 to Y2.5 million worth of products yearly, mainly to hospitals. In maintaining a supply of almost any product on the market, the government agency has some advantage over the more than two dozen private enterprises in the county that now also sell modern drugs, whose stocks are smaller and where a customer may find items temporarily out of stock or not carried at all. By the same token, the products are much cheaper in the private stores. In Chinese herbs, there is a very active free-market trade, with hospitals among the buyers as well as physicians in private practice.

The shortage in rural areas of physicians with a high degree of technical competency was hardly remarkable. Chinese physicians are no different from their counterparts around the world. They prefer to work in the cities, in comfortable surroundings, with the potential of professional and monetary reward. In China, regular medical college graduates have until recently generally been easily able to find positions in any one of hundreds of urban hospitals, clinics, and research facilities. With the turnout of medical schools increasing, some graduates have joined county facilities in recent years; but perceived hardships still limit willingness to work at the xiang level. If at least some medical school graduates could be persuaded to serve the village population in xiang centers, the possibility of early diagnosis and treatment of infectious disease cases would be greatly enhanced. With good public health training, these graduates might even begin to think in terms of practicing community medicine.

WESTERN MEDICAL EDUCATION SEEN
THROUGH THE "OPEN-DOOR"

As I had long since come to realize, this issue of the quality of personnel—the largest area of vulnerability in our rural health service—could not be solved without rendering our regular medical school graduates more community-minded. This is the reason for the intensification of my interest in medical education and for eagerness of my response when the Ministry of Health, acting in accord with the "open-door" policy, made it possible for me to go abroad to study patterns of medical education in Canada and the United States in 1979.

My views had begun to be of some interest to the authorities, and in early 1979 I had been called to Beijing to attend an official seminar on medical education and public health education. Then, in the fall of the same year, the Ministry of Health delegated me to travel to North America to study the medical school curricula in Canada and the United States with respect to how they could be adapted for use in our own country. On my return, I prepared a report with some recommendations to the Ministry of Health. The next year, on another study trip, I visited the Institute of Rural Reconstruction established in the Philippines in 1967 by James Y. C. Yen, my long-time friend from Dingxian days who had founded and directed the Mass Education Movement in prerevolutionary China.

On the 1979 trip to North America, the first stop, in Canada, entailed visits to the Medical School of the University of Toronto, in Toronto, Ontario and the McMaster University Medical School in Hamilton, Ontario. My brother, a university teacher, met me at the airport after a journey that, compared with previous Pacific crossings, had been very brief. In 1946 it had taken three days by air to reach the Western coast of North America; this time it had taken fewer than twenty hours.

While favorably impressed by the Medical School at the University of Toronto, especially by its research in immunology and biomedical engineering, I found the visit to the Medical School of McMaster University more rewarding because of its innovative approach to teaching. There was a great deal of creative thinking behind the planned program. For example, emphasis on self-study, using available resources, was begun at admission. Students and teachers worked in close relationship. Public service, rather than personal reward, was stressed. All in all, it seemed a good model for China.

In the United States, I was eager to see what developments had taken place in the twenty-five years since relations between our two countries had ended. At Harvard University, I visited the Schools of Public Health and Medicine. The faculty had increased enormously, and its interests seemed to revolve less around challenging the students than in generating papers on subjects of high academic interest. Many research topics, as far as I saw, had no connection with major health problems. An encouraging sign at the medical school was the development of a new department of family medicine, with a relatively generalized focus. As to efforts to instill any interest in public health in the students, however, I was not aware of much.

With one exception, other schools I visited seemed to have changed greatly in size but to have changed their teaching methods, educational objectives, and field training activities very little. There was no evidence that the teaching of preventive medicine and public health was respected in the medical schools; possibly the separation of teaching of clinical medicine and public health contributed to this situation. Instruction seemed to be less generally characterized by intellectual stimulation than by reliance on audiovisual aids. It was gratifying to note at Cornell University Medical School, however, that the students were being asked to do field surveys.

The exceptional school was the Medical School of the University of Missouri in Kansas City, which, under a pilot program, was accepting high-school students for admission and in its coursework was emphasizing a population-based approach to medical studies. The director, E. Grey Dimond, M.D., a cardiologist, impressed me as a talented administrator.

In the light of this trip, I felt that the United States was not doing much through its medical education system to imbue its students with a sense of public service and a responsibility to think beyond individual casework and specialized research. I regret that in the medical schools I visited I did not see departments of public health as strong as that of the PUMC in the era of leadership by John B. Grant half a century ago. The schools of public health that I visited in the eastern part of the United States had become research institutions where technology and publication of technical papers generally dictated educational direction.

PART III

Sharing Insights

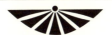

7

Reflections on the Health Experience

All told, my life and work as a modern physician and medical educator span well over fifty years, during which time my primary consideration has focused on community medicine and public health. Even after that long interval, I have no final answer to the question that has absorbed me persistently: "How best can we introduce scientific medicine into an untutored population and make it take root there for the benefit of the common people?"

The course of my life has, nevertheless, yielded a number of insights that I believe should be shared with other persons in medical education, community medicine, and public health around the world. Those working in developing countries may find the Chinese experience in organizing rural health care to be particularly relevant.

A DEVELOPING NATION AND ITS HEALTH CARE SYSTEM

Before sharing those insights, however, it might be well to point out certain assumptions that underlie my thinking about health care delivery in developing countries and, for that matter, health care in any society, for those beliefs shape the specific judgments at which I have arrived.

The first of these is the conviction that the strength of any nation lies in its common people, and that the best possible health care, therefore, should be available to the population as a whole, not just to a privileged few. I have the deepest respect for the common people of my own country—most of whom are village-dwelling farmers—and see them as the bedrock of our nation. Their agricultural capacity and their fortitude in adversity contribute greatly to national stability.

The belief that the common people are the bedrock of the nation, anchored in ancient Chinese teaching, has been revitalized and given new meaning under CCP rule. The philosophy of hard work and equality has already yielded better lives for the people. Since liberation in 1949, economic well-being has increased, educational opportunity has expanded, and for many, living conditions have improved. Combined with greatly improved health care and the curtailment of population growth, these developments have brought a remarkable decline in mortality and increase in life expectancy.

The common people, I suspect, are the wellspring of national vitality in many other countries besides China, especially those whose economies are also based on agriculture and whose populations consist predominantly of village-dwelling farmers. Some developing countries, as well as some highly developed nations, however, may fail to see a correlation between the national interest and the well-being of the grass-roots population. Promoting public health in such societies may be an especially difficult task.

A second belief that is fundamental in my personal thinking about health care is that medicine based on scientific principles is inherently superior to any system that lacks that foundation. This statement in no way is intended to denigrate the traditional medicine of my own country or that of any other. Indigenous Chinese medicine, for instance, has provided medical relief to countless millions of persons over the ages, withstanding the test of time, and offering sustained evidence that many of its remedies indeed have some degree of efficacy. The same is apt to be true, to varying degrees, of the indigenous medicines of other countries.

Nevertheless, in my view, because it is formulated and systematized in accordance with verifiable general laws, scientific medicine enjoys an unsurpassable margin of superiority over any competing system of medicine. In the substance of traditional Chinese medicine, for example, there is nothing comparable to the scientifi-

cally informed explanations of anatomy, physiology, and patho-
genesis that are basic to modern medicine.

In methodology and application as well, the differences are no
less significant. The criteria of diagnosis, rationale for treatment,
methods of physical and laboratory examination, and analysis of
laboratory results found in modern medicine simply have no counterpart in our traditional system. As to application, the vantage
ground is clear. Concern with health protection and improvement
is all but self-defeating without attention to preventive measures,
which can have a crucial impact on health levels. For evidence, one
has only to consider the contribution of China's mass-immuniza-
tion campaigns to the dramatic decrease in mortality in our country
since 1949. Yet, whereas scientific medicine assigns some importance to preventive measures, traditional medicine in practice ne-
glects them almost entirely.

In passing, it must be recognized, of course, that scientific medicine, too, has limitations. In any event, regardless of what treatment is used, a patient's successful recovery may at times be attributed as much to nature's intervention as to the ministrations of the
physician. We have no way of knowing all that is involved in the
natural course of development of an illness. Getting the public to
understand the complexity of cause-and-effect relationships is a
problem in medicine, as elsewhere. Notwithstanding the limitations of scientific medicine, however, I remain convinced that its
application to our national health problems is more in the interest
of the people than undue support and expansion of our traditional
system.

For those who hope for growing confidence in scientific medicine and its broadened application for the public benefit in any
country where traditional medicine has deep roots, time and effort
are required in order to achieve organizational change. Meanwhile
it is up to us to help to promote scientific understanding throughout the general population and to advocate qualitative improvement in modern medical training.

Like my commitment to the welfare of the common people and
my conviction of the relative superiority of scientific medicine, the
third and final premise of my medical philosophy derives from the
experiences of childhood and youth. Since a young age I have
taken it for granted that no worthwhile national goal can be

achieved without attention to education. This is no less true in medicine and public health than in any other realm. Anyone interested in seeing the further application of scientific medical knowledge in any country, developing or otherwise, cannot escape responsibility as an educator.

This responsibility assumes special importance with respect to the villagers and nomadic peoples of developing countries. Given the educational levels of modern, industrialized societies, it can fairly safely be assumed that the majority of their populations have at least a fundamental store of scientific knowledge. By extension, therefore, we can further assume that they have been at least minimally exposed to the idea that infectious disease is caused by microorganisms that enter, grow, and multiply in the body, and that many diseases are transmitted by contagion.

In developing countries, however, we can make no such assumption. As is widely recognized, their populations are generally partially or wholly uninformed about basic scientific matters. Many villagers around the world have no idea how infection is contracted or disease transmitted. In fact, illness is often attributed to the work of malevolent spirits. As long as this notion prevails among villagers, we cannot expect them to be concerned about maintaining personal cleanliness or taking aseptic precautions in their daily lives. They will simply adhere to their old ways.

Thus, regardless of the immense challenges that confront health professionals in Third World countries in trying to treat the sick, it is important, at least initially, that they spare some time for health education efforts. Pressures from other directions must be balanced by the need to develop a scientifically informed population made up of men, women, and children who have at least some elementary understanding of scientific principles. Otherwise we can anticipate that efforts to protect and improve health through the application of scientific medicine will have only a short-term and superficial impact.

This was the rationale for the progressive action that several other PUMC students and I took in establishing the *Binying Weekly*, the newspaper health supplement that we wrote and published as medical students in Beijing. Our aim was to make the educated newspaper readers of the city better informed in health matters and to encourage them to press the warlord regimes for improved health care. Medical students today have no less a responsibility to educate the public, and their teachers, in turn, should encourage them along these lines. The education of the public in health matters is one avenue through which community-oriented physicians can discharge their professional obligations.

THE PROCESS OF RURAL HEALTH
DEVELOPMENT: LESSONS FROM CHINA

Making modern medical care accessible to the entire population of a developing country, and fostering its acceptance and use, cannot be accomplished overnight. The process requires time and patience. It implies fundamental change in the way people think and behave as well as the education and training of scientific personnel, and the organization of a health system, in which those persons can function effectively.

Six somewhat overlapping stages seem to be involved in the process. First, an appropriate relationship must be worked out with whatever indigenous medical system exists. Next, it is necessary to identify and educate a vanguard of young medical scientists and to imbue them with idealism and enthusiasm to undertake a difficult pioneering venture. Prepared for the task, the new leaders must produce, through trial and error, a model of health care suited to the needs and resources of that particular society. Foreign models are usually unsuitable, at least in part. The government must lend strong support, preferably before, and certainly after, the model has been developed, so that modern medical care can be made accessible in all parts of the country within the framework of an integrated, nationwide system of health care. Besides facilitating the countrywide establishment of the health network, the government must provide initial and continuing education for technical and support personnel at all levels. Finally, refinement and improvement of the system must be fostered through an ongoing two-way exchange of ideas, knowledge, and experience with other countries engaged in comparable efforts.

Scientific medicine was first introduced into our society over an urban bridgehead from the West well over a century ago. Thus China has already moved through many of these stages. Perhaps it is not too early to gain from our experience, enabling us to enlarge on the promising results for better health and long life that we have already achieved. There may be lessons also for other predominantly agricultural countries, whose young leaders are just now confronting issues and challenges that our leadership faced on the eve of our liberation, now nearly 40 years ago.

DEALING WITH TRADITIONAL MEDICINE

In rural China, traditional medicine remains very powerful. Traditional hospitals and clinics are crowded with patients, traditional practitioners are prospering, and the farmers generally use more herbs than standardized pharmaceuticals. Traditional medicine, along with scientific medicine, receives strong support from the central government, and many high officials seem to be persuaded that traditional medicine offers benefits possibly not found in a scientific medical system.

One might well ask how this could be possible. Scientific medicine had been introduced into China more than a century earlier and had quickly obtained a firm footing in urban areas. Moreover, intellectual and reformist currents that swept our country in the 1920s had vaulted science and scientific thinking to a pinnacle of approbation among influential intellectuals of the day, who saw its potential for bettering human life as almost boundless.

A century, in terms of our country's long and complex past, is a relatively brief time span, however, and for the answer one has to reach much more deeply into the ages. Chinese as a people have a strong sense of history. We cherish our ancient cultural heritage and value traditional medicine as a component of that heritage. Moreover, many, if not most, of us have full confidence in the time-tested measures of medical relief that traditional medicine affords. In rural areas, this confidence may be especially engrained, associated as it was for centuries with the endorsement of respected imperial scholars.

The power of traditional medicine in the contemporary scene is, in part, explicable in these terms. Probably still more important however, is the lingering effect of the century after century during which its scholar-physician practitioners ranked in the highest strata of society and enjoyed the confidence and support of the

imperial rulers. The social and political influence of traditional practitioners in urban China today mirrors that historical position.

Ironically, the outspoken minority of modern physicians who, in
the early twentieth century, campaigned to have traditional medicine legally abolished suceeded only in increasing its public support. The failure of their strategy reflected a blindness to important
cultural realities. Unlike modern medicine, traditional medicine
had been developed in Chinese soil by Chinese physicians, who
shared a philosophical and intellectual background with the highest officials. Among a people who revered their millennia-old civilization and culture and respected the wisdom of classical scholars,
that was more than sufficient to ensure its survival. Had modern
medicine advocates steered a more moderate course, traditional
medicine would very likely be far less powerful than it is today,
and the circumstances would have been more conducive to the
diffusion of scientific medicine in our society.

Those who had tried to ban traditional medicine had miscalcu-
lated both the political resources of the urban-based scholars and
the depth of public attachment to traditional medicine. More explic-
itly stated, perhaps, the idea was unrealistic. Advocates of abolition entirely ignored the attitudes and circumstances of the villagers, who formed the majority of the population. The peasants by
and large lacked access to any other kind of medicine, but,
tradition-bound as they were, they were unlikely to have tried it
even if they had had access.

Although modern medical care is widely available in rural China
today, attempts to prevent the general population from using traditional medicine would be as ill-advised in the late 1980s as they
were then, especially in areas where well-trained modern physicians are rare. Traditional medicine is much more acceptable to
Chinese of all walks of life than is scientific medicine because it is
more closely linked to our thinking and philosophy of life. People
believe in it, and when they are ill, many, if not most, people want
to consult a traditional practitioner, not a modern physician. In our
country, modern medicine will supplant traditional medicine only
gradually and slowly, possibly only among distant generations,
and then only as a result of careful scientific education and demonstration of its efficacy.

The confrontation between scientific and indigenous medicine in our country, then, has perhaps been especially instructive. As we saw in the chapters on preliberation China, the introduction of science, including scientific medicine, into a largely uneducated population is never an easy matter, especially when its indigenous medicine is widely endorsed and culturally valued. In any modernizing society, social and intellectual, as well as technical, difficulties always exist. A scientific mentality must be encouraged in the general population. Where there is strong political support for traditional medicine, as in our country, the problem becomes even more complicated. Tolerance toward traditional medicine may be the wisest choice. Meanwhile efforts should be made to apply scientific methods to the study of any medications or procedures used by indigenous medicine that seem to be useful.

Notwithstanding previous problems, in China today relations between the two systems of medicine are cordial; practitioners respect each other. Thoughtful minds on both sides recognize that to the extent that it interferes with health care delivery, it is a waste of time to dwell on differences. The important point is to develop a health care system that works as a united force to improve the health and prolong the lives of the people.

While it is pointless to dwell on differences, it may not be very realistic to think in terms of "integration." Perhaps in some countries it might be possible to integrate scientific medicine and the indigenous medical system with beneficial effect. In our case, in fact, some highly placed party and government officials have advocated that idea. Seemingly, they are convinced that, in such a synthesis, traditional medicine would play a significant role, given its time-tested theories, abundant clinical experience, and attraction as a subject of study by Western medical specialists. Recently, however, other officials have expressed a less sanguine point of view, cautioning that in an integrated discipline, traditional medicine might actually be absorbed and disappear.

Personally, I am compelled to ask myself what "integration" might mean when so little common ground is shared. Modern medicine had its beginnings in Europe after the Renaissance in the work of such great men as Andreas Vesalius in the sixteenth century, whose work—based on a precise record of observed facts, rather than opinion and speculation—laid the groundwork for scientific anatomical observation.

Traditional medicine is by no means entirely unscientific; it is partly the result of a large amount of experience, just as is modern medicine. But it has no such foundation in scientific observation. Common ground is also lacking in such other areas as methods of examination, consideration of side effects, and attention to prevention. For all these reasons, there will always be areas where physicians on one side or the other will have difficulty understanding each other.

We can see the consequences of the lack of shared ground in the dilemma in which some of our traditional medical students apparently find themselves. Their course of study is challenging. Nowadays they are required to study scientific subjects, including anatomy and physiology. Beginning with the third year, they work under the guidance of an experienced practitioner, learning case by case, through clinical experience, examining patients, and seeing the effects of the drugs they use. Familiarizing themselves with the immense number of Chinese drugs during this period is a formidable challenge in itself. The student must also, of course, become informed about the underlying theories of traditional treatment; traditional medical texts are by no means easy to read. The meaning of passages containing an admixture of description of empirical observations and metaphysical theory may be quite obscure.

All this is challenging enough. Additionally, however, students must somehow correlate the traditional theories with scientific observations and explanations to which they have been exposed during their first two years of study. This can lead to problems in understanding the reason for the diagnosis and treatment prescribed.

Under such circumstances, interesting young people in both traditional and modern medicine concurrently can be very difficult. The teacher trying to make traditional and modern medicine compatible, either in theoretical discussion or in practical work, faces a real challenge. I personally have taken short courses in traditional medicine, and because of my background in modern medicine—which, needless to say, is quite different from that of a traditional practioner, the more I studied it, the more confused I became.

At present it is difficult to predict the outcome of our educational program and activities designed to promote integration. It does, however, seem quite apparent that neither political authority nor popular response alone can bring it about. Possibly for many years to come the two types of practitioner will be working on their own basis, side by side, each receiving government support. Meanwhile, whatever else may be said, our solution to the coexistence of two medicines is uniquely Chinese and has produced a uniquely Chinese health system.

Before leaving the subject of traditional medicine, it might be noted that Chinese research institutes have given high priority to research on drugs, which is not surprising given the historic tendency in our country to regard the dispensation of drugs as the essence of medicine as a discipline. Priority research areas include cancer, retinal disease, and fertility, with the focus on finding drugs that have never been known to the outside world and that would produce an effect not obtainable in scientific medicine. A global breakthrough in medical research would be a source of great national pride to our country, as to any other country.

Developing Pioneer Leadership

The introduction of scientific medicine into societies undergoing modernization requires dedicated pioneer leadership and at least a handful of gifted teachers to bring it along. On the basis of my experience, in fact, I would say that the nurturing of innovative and idealistic leadership in the first generation of newly trained modern medical scientists is crucial to future public health development in any country. In this context, the inspiration of a few good teachers to even a minority of students can make a critical difference, especially if those teachers are concerned with broad issues affecting health rather than with specific clinical interests.

Consider, for example, John B. Grant, the physician who was for many years the Rockefeller Foundation representative in the Far East and concurrently the head of the Department of Health at the Peking Union Medical College (PUMC), which I attended. To me and many of my classmates, Grant was a crucially important source of direction. Most PUMC students tended to regard public health courses as the least welcome elements in the curriculum. Grant accepted that view as a challenge and went on to develop an innovative public health program involving intensive field study that caught the imaginations of many participants. His success lay in confronting students with the scope of health problems in the general population and relating this to the capacity of scientific medicine to alleviate them.

Under Grant, students who might otherwise have entered private practice became interested in the diffusion of modern medicine for a common good. I, for example, at Grant's recommendation, became health director for the Mass Education Movement (MEM) at Dingxian in the 1930s. In subsequently pioneering the organization of our country's first systematic rural health care organization in that county, I was never unaware of Grant's influence on my thinking.

He convinced me that insight and experience gained in field training is as important a component of public health studies as is substantive knowledge acquired in the classroom, if not more important. I quickly came to see, too, that knowledge, however gained, is to be valued not for its content, but for its applicability to the problems at hand. The rewards of pursuing knowledge for its own sake must be left to others.

This exposure later brought me to realize the merit of the PUMC decision to use English as the language of instruction, rather than Chinese, as was done at a number of missionary medical schools. I am convinced that the use of English as the teaching vehicle greatly enhanced the value of our education. Taught in Chinese, we would have acquired the substantive knowledge necessary to practice modern medicine as well as the clinical skills. Our scientific training would have been complete. We would, however, have been left with no real sense of the intellectual and philosophical underpinnings of Western medicine, nor would Grant or other teachers really have exercised much influence on our personal spiritual and moral perceptions. This humanistic side of our education was important; for the education of a modern medical student should involve far more than the mere transfer of substantive knowledge of clinical skills. Medicine is an art, as well as a science.

Admittedly, there was a negative side to this issue. The use of English presented difficulties on both sides, and more than one potentially excellent candidate was excluded from the PUMC program because of the language barrier.

By singling out one teacher and that teacher's influence, I mean in no way to diminish the general overall value of the education we received at the PUMC and the contribution of the institution as a whole on my thinking. That was of crucial importance in our development as pioneering national leaders in health. Many of our medical professors were outstanding specialists in one clinical field or another, and our training under their guidance was invaluable.

The insistence on high standards of medical excellence benefited not only the PUMC students themselves but also other Chinese medical schools whose more modest institutional administrations struggled to emulate the model. As a result, over a period of several decades the poor standards of many struggling missionary, Japanese, and government-run Chinese medical schools gradually improved to a marked degree.

Fulfillment of the Rockefeller Foundation goal of providing medical leadership for China had begun as soon as the first students left the walled campus in Beijing to pursue their careers. The PUMC produced just over 300 graduates in twenty-five years, but the influence of those few was far out of proportion to their number, and a majority of graduates figured importantly in public health, medical education, and medical administration in our country over the next half-century and beyond.

Over the years the reputation of the PUMC came to be based largely on its contributions to scientific research and clinical medical education, its input to national development not going much beyond significant accomplishment in these spheres. As to the contribution made by the few faculty members who interested students in tackling the ordinary and immense medical problems of the general population, and who imbued them with high ideals and a spirit of resourcefulness in so doing, little was said. In the long run, however, the role of the PUMC in educating public health leaders may have been in every sense as important to China, if not more so, than its role in developing clinical specialists, research scientists, and professors of medicine.

Fifty years ago ignorance and superstition shaped the lives of the Chinese peasantry, just as it does the lives of rural inhabitants of many developing countries today. Educational opportunity was lacking for most urban inhabitants as well, and the population of the cities, if somewhat better educated, was no less superstition-ridden. Until this medieval mentality was replaced with some un-

derstanding of science, and until most Chinese more fully appreciated the need for cleanliness and sanitation, not much progress
could be expected in diffusing modern medicine throughout the
society.

The fact that a minority of PUMC recognized popular ignorance
of scientific principles as an obstacle to health improvement and
tried to provide a remedy and proceeded to concern themselves
with the medical realities in rural areas is, I believe, part of the
special legacy of the PUMC to our country. Unless there had been
at least a few graduates prepared to undertake public health work
in rural China, under difficult conditions—and willing to sacrifice
their own personal and monetary gain and to persist, despite the
often frustratingly slow pace of change—rural health services
would have improved far less rapidly. Social change in every society requires leaders with creative ideas and high ideals.

Notwithstanding the significant contribution of the PUMC to
China, a few aspects of its policy, even for that time, seem to have
been less than closely attuned to the needs of the country. For
example, the PUMC gave meticulous attention to the advanced
technical training of a few nurses. In itself, this was a valuable
undertaking. What China really needed at that time, however, was
also an army of practical nurses who could do bedside work, train
other practical nurses, and imbue in the patients some practices
that could enable them to improve their standards of cleanliness
and comfort.

An elite institution can be an effective educational tool, as the
PUMC clearly showed. It provided its students with many advantages, including, most conspicuously, but not exclusively, a fundamental appreciation of science and the scientific method, and a
solid grounding in the disciplines concerned with sickness and
health. It set an admirable level of technical standards.

The real problems with an approach that emphasized technical
excellence to such a degree, however, is that it risks the deprivation
of any developing country of the very kind of physicians it most
needs, dedicated innovators and idealists willing to roll up their
shirt sleeves and work at the grass-roots level, attacking problems
in the soil where they exist.

Had its students lived under conditions that were more in keeping with those of the surrounding population, rather than on a

level with those of the elite group in a highly industrialized Western country, perhaps a larger number of graduates would have been prepared to serve their country. As it was, some graduates, accustomed to the lifestyle they had enjoyed as students, left China for the West. Of those who remained, very few were willing to live under uncomfortable conditions among the rural peasants.

Another observation based on the PUMC experience that might be useful to an institution of its type in a developing country today concerns the role of indigenous leadership in institutional policymaking. Although China in the 1920s had its own modern-educated class, input from the Chinese side into PUMC decisions was seldom encouraged. In developing countries today, where educated and experienced leadership is apt to be in short supply, it may be particularly important that country nationals be given an opportunity to participate in policymaking along with the foreign advisors. This will not only provide experience for some people but will also facilitate integration of the institution with the society at large.

Whatever the value of an elite educational institution in a developing country may be, it should not be perceived as the sole source of competent leadership, either for the organization of health care or for any other modernization goal. Able leaders are to be found everywhere, not just in a small pool of exceptionally gifted students, or of students who have particular social origins, a special language capability, or a certain level of formal education.

I remember once at Dingxian expressing concern to Andrija Stampar, the public health leader from Yugoslavia who was visiting our site, as to where I would find competent people to work with me in the districtwide health system we were establishing. "What?" Stampar asked. "You have 400,000 people here, and no leaders?"

His question was appropriate. It may be that too often we think in terms of stereotypes and have fixed conceptions of leadership, blinding us to its existence when we find it other than where we expect it.

Competitive examinations for university entrance, for example, or rigid academic standards often serve a useful purpose; at times, however, they may deprive a society of the talent it sorely needs. Bright, energetic, and able young people, regardless of their personal or educational circumstances, have something to contribute to pioneer leadership in health development. In addition, we may have to uncover their innate capacities by the simple process of giving them a chance to show what they can do, weeding out the less competent through trial and error. There should be more than one fixed path to leadership.

DIRECTING CHANGE THROUGH EXPERIMENTATION

In the late nineteenth and early twentieth centuries, China theoretically accepted the Western pattern of private medical practice as appropriate for its own use only to realize that, whereas this health system might suit the needs and resources of a modern, industrialized society, it was not compatible with Chinese conditions. In the midtwentieth century China once again turned to a foreign model, emulating Soviet patterns in medical and public health education and in institutional organization for research. An alternative in both cases would have been to work out our own models, or to modify the borrowed ones, in accordance with social and economic conditions specific for our country.

Cost was a major factor in the inappropriateness of the Western system of medical practice for China. Outside support had been required to establish and maintain its urban-centered hospitals and clinics, and, to any thinking person, it was clear that should that external support ever be withdrawn, the system was likely to collapse. Moreover, its philosophical basis engendered wasteful competition among individual physicians rather than a collective response to the overwhelming medical problems of a modernizing country.

More importantly, Western medical practice served only a privileged minority of urban Chinese, largely ignoring the needs for medical attention among the millions upon millions of peasants in the countryside, who constituted the vast majority of the population. In many rural districts there were no medical facilities of any kind; in some there were even no traditional practitioners. After 1928 the Guomindang party somewhat succeeded in organizing urban health administrations and establishing a number of urban

hospitals and clinics; however, rural needs were generally neglected. By and large, the villagers remained deadlocked in the grip
of poverty, disease, and ignorance of a feudal era.

There were, during the 1920s and 1930s, however, a few privately
assisted groups working in areas of rural China, experimenting with
various innovative measures to enhance the lives of the peasants.
The Mass Education Movement (MEM) based at Dingxian—with
which I served as health director for more than seven years—was
one of these. As we have seen in chapter 3, it was this organization
that provided me with the opportunity I had been seeking since
medical school, namely, to experiment with a health system to reach
the peasants.

Working with the MEM offered several advantages that may not
always be available to developing country health personnel fram-
ing programs in their own countries. First, at the MEM we were
not trying to deal with the health problems of the community in
isolation. Rather, we were part of a closely correlated four-point
program of socioeconomic change. Education, agricultural techniques, farm credit, and civic training were simultaneously receiving close attention; for even at that early time the MEM leadership
had already recognized that the roots of rural problems are inter-
woven and that coordinated programs for socioeconomic improvement need to be developed. The quality of preventive medicine
and of available treatment is just one of the influences affecting the
health of a population.

Another advantage I enjoyed as health director was that I had a
great deal of autonomy and was able to work systematically and
without undue haste. The MEM was a privately organized group,
and as such could offer its administrative staff greater leverage for
experimentation than a government agency can usually afford, as
private groups are accountable to the public or the government
only in the broadest sense. In testing some rather unusual ideas
through trial and error, therefore, I was relative unhampered by
external constraints or by any pressure to come up with a quick
answer. This was important, for a model must be tested as it is
devised. Components may not work and will need to be adjusted
before the model is adapted by administrators in other parts of the
country.

Freedom to experiment and time to formulate viable solutions had permitted us to develop a system that received global recognition for its resourceful solutions to knotty problems. Since then, some of our ideas have been disseminated around the world and after some fifty years may no longer seem quite so innovative. At that time and place, however—Dingxian China in the 1930s, we broke ground in many respects. Of our basic working ideas, four were particularly noteworthy.

First, we based our approach to health care on local needs and conditions. Rather than coming in with any preconceived ideas, we conducted our own statistical surveys as a basis for planning and consulted with local community leaders to obtain their ideas of the major problems in the district. The notion of taking surveys as part of a planning procedure was virtually nonexistent in our country at that time.

Second, we devised a system that was locally affordable, diminishing the economic barrier that previously had rendered modern medical care inaccessible to most villagers. We did this by basing plans on the collective use of the very small funds available in the village, amounting to less than U.S.$0.10 per capita annually.

Third, we constructed a bridge over which modern medicine as practiced in China's larger cities was carried to the rural areas. Student doctors and nurses from the leading urban hospitals of China came to the Dingxian field training site, where they saw and treated rural patients who heretofore had relied solely on untrained village practitioners.

Fourth, and last, we insisted on community responsibility for the operation and continued effectiveness of the system. In our physicians, nurses, and health workers, as well as among the villagers themselves, we tried to foster habits of cooperation for good community health, such as the early reporting of infectious diseases and the encouragement of a sanitary environment. Beyond this, we made local community organizations responsible for the ethical and responsible conduct of local health workers.

BUILDING THE INFRASTRUCTURE

All these attributes of the Dingxian model were noteworthy. As its originator, however, I believe that its most critical attribute was its emphasis on systematic procedures and careful regulation of technical responsibility at each level. I am a strong believer in effective organization, and it is this aspect of the Dingxian model that I hope health workers from other countries will find of particular interest. We might have offered modern medical care of sorts to the villagers under several different circumstances, but the high quality of care to which they gained access was possible only because systematic organization was fundamental to our approach.

At Dingxian, health care was rendered through a three-tiered system of village, subdistrict, and district units. Different responsibilities were assigned to each type of unit, in accordance with the different degrees of training of the senior staff at each level. The marked difference in the technical competency of those in charge at each level ensured control of quality.

The system allowed not only for effective collaboration of all levels but also for careful supervision up and down the line. No one was expected or permitted to undertake tasks beyond one's technical capability, and staff at each level respected the superior knowledge and skill of those of higher grade.

From what I have seen in Shifang County in the mid-1980s, I could imagine that some barefoot doctors today have come to regard themselves as more competent than the secondary medical school graduates in charge of the xiang health clinics. This is an unfortunate situation and places the patient in an awkward position. At Dingxian, however, we had been able to circumvent this difficulty through a policy of graduated responsibility based on marked differences in the degree of technical training among personnel at each level.

Our system at Dingxian was built from the bottom upward. By this I mean that we used the least trained workers in the villages, better trained persons at the intermediate level, and the best trained at the county level. We trained our own village-based workers, giving them only simple instruction in health fundamentals, first aid, and techniques of immunization, and impressing on them the necessity of referring patients to the subdistrict unit for early diagnosis of serious illness or for further treatment. Each subdistrict unit was supervised by a graduate physician, who managed a junior staff, while I headed the district unit, whose senior staff were the most technically competent people in the system.

Dingxian was built from the bottom upward also in the sense

that we based our approach on what our surveys and our informants identified as the major health needs of the community, rather than coming in with any prefixed idea of how our system would operate. I am convinced that this is the logical starting point. After all, if many people believe or want something, there is considerable social force behind that collective opinion, and in trying to respond to the need, you will get cooperation. When you start at the top and work downward, as the missionaries tried to do in our country, you often find yourself dealing with relatively few individuals and relatively rare conditions while neglecting the chronic problems of the community at large.

In a three-tiered modern health care system such as we had at Dingxian, the technical training of the key people at the middle level must be unarguably superior to that of the health workers in the villages. Otherwise, one of two circumstances will develop, neither one of which is conducive to the spread of scientific medicine. Villagers may either fall back on traditional practitioners or they will rely on barefoot doctors who may not be sufficiently trained or supervised to provide quality care. Villagers will either develop confidence in modern-trained sources of relief or rely on the village health workers to do more than they have been properly trained to do, and the quality of care will suffer.

To anyone attempting to establish a rural health system in a developing country, I would recommend, on the basis of our experience, recruiting for local leaders in the existing community organizations and preparing them to do the elementary tasks that are most needed in that community. These needs will vary from place to place, particularly in an immense and diversified country such as ours. In one area, for example, potable water may be a priority issue and in another area, the control of malaria. The safest way to determine those needs is by consulting local leaders and by conducting preliminary surveys. Needs should be identified on where they actually emerge, not out of textbooks.

Health workers who live in the villages are essential to the maintenance of quality care, but if their training is minimal, their services should be limited to immunization and first aid work. Learning to use a few instruments is a rather simple matter; however, disciplined scientific thinking comes much harder, and this is why diagnostic responsibilities should be reserved to those with sound scientific knowledge and more advanced clinical training. To make such persons available to seriously ill village patients obviously requires that the intermediate and higher levels of the infrastructure be organized as soon as possible after the village health workers have been selected and trained.

No matter how suitable a model for rural health services may seem through experimentation, no one will gain much unless the government is active in extending it. Our experience under Guomindang officialdom taught us that. Party officials had recommended in 1934 that the Dingxian model be adopted throughout China, but there had been little follow-up, not so much because of the outbreak of war in 1937 as because of lack of genuine commitment on the part of the goverment to addressing rural needs.

Even for a decade after liberation in 1949, little was done in rural health other than construction of a few county hospitals and clinics and the dispatch of mobile units to distant areas. Once CCP Chairman Mao Zedong became disillusioned with urban intellectuals, however, and criticized the Ministry of Health as the "ministry for influential people," rural health development accelerated rapidly. Without his strong backing, it is most unlikely that the massive and abrupt expansion of rural health care service and the recruitment of the required personnel that this entailed would have occurred. Rural health development in other countries today probably also demands strong input from the central government.

The buildup of the county health system of three levels in rural China was both directly and indirectly based on preliberation experience. Authorities drew heavily on the Dingxian model. They did, however, differentiate from it at points where they evidently thought that adherence was inessential or impossible. For example, lower priorities were assigned to development of adjunct training programs and attention to quality control through integration and careful gradation of responsibility.

The remarkable achievement realized from the expansion of the infrastructure in our country was the astonishing amount of prevention work that was done within the villages and by persons who lived right in the villages. This, again, reinforces the importance of the lowest level of the three-tiered system. By 1959, in many areas of the country, plague, smallpox, kala azar, typhus, and relapsing fever had all been brought under control. Environmental sanitation improved as a result of mass health campaigns to promote cleanliness and eradicate insects. In the 1960s, malaria and schistosomiasis were great reduced. Later attacks were launched on smallpox, measles, diphtheria, whooping cough, typhoid, and poliomyelitis.

The point that warrants emphasis is that the work was done right in the villages. In my view, there is no hope of controlling infectious diseases without such a contingent of health workers who do actually live in the village, regardless of how high a priority central authorities assign that aim. Effective immunization cannot be accomplished merely by sending in mobile teams. Farmers often cannot comply with their schedules and are neither able nor willing to bring their children to mobile stations in sufficient numbers. One may elicit a 50 to 60 percent response at most, but not the 90 percent necessary for effective control.

Providing Trained Personnel

In the fifth step of building a nationwide health care system, personnel must be developed to staff the expanding infrastructure. Ideally, the infrastructure develops only as swiftly as personnel can be trained to meet requirements. In reality, of course, this is seldom possible, and compromises may have to be made.

Rapid extension often means the lowering of personnel standards and the inadequacy of facilities. There can be no guarantee of quality in service or teaching. Qualified personnel cannot be properly recruited and trained in a short time, and any system built on unqualified personnel may defeat the purpose of rendering good care to the general population. A government is generally aware of the disadvantages associated with rapid expansion, but usually for political reasons, large-scale extension with inadequate personnel, equipment, and financial support is carried out at the expense of quality. The only remedy thereafter is to improve the quality of personnel by local training.

Such firsthand opportunities as I have had to observe rural medical care corroborate my belief in the importance of field training and the local training school for health for personnel in our country. In Shifang County I have personally seen a number of instances where an unfortunate situation might have been avoided if the physician in attendance had received better training. There was, for example, a patient with shoulder pain whose shoulder was dislocated by the examining barefoot doctor. Another patient with a fracture paid for a costly x-ray that was essentially worthless because it had been taken by an untrained medical assistant who did not know how to use the equipment properly.

Even in relatively routine situations, it would be helpful if barefoot doctors had more training, and consequently more confidence in their own competency. For example, a barefoot doctor, unsure of what is causing the cough and fever of a small child, and without anyone with more advanced training to turn too, as a precaution may prescribe penicillin when, in fact, the simple suggestion of bedrest and plenty of fluids would have served just as well. In such a situation, the mother of the precious "one child" will almost certainly spend her money for the expensive, but needless, prescription.

The difficulty of doing this well in China is very great, however, in part because the county training schools for health schools must deal with people whose educational backgrounds are so extremely limited. What we greatly need, therefore, is some pioneer effort to show the sizable positive impact that a really effective county training school program can have on rural health.

Benefiting from Foreign Contact

In the sixth and final phase, responsible health leaders must take deliberate steps to constantly refine and improve the health care system, relying not only on their own ideas but also on fresh inspiration from outside. If the doors are left open to foreign contact, health administrators, medical educators, physicians, nurses, and other health professionals from other parts of the world can be a rich source of innovative ideas in a two-way flow that benefits both sides.

Free exchange of ideas and knowledge, as I learned as a child, leads to mutual understanding and appreciation. This is a principle of human life equally applicable to relationships between individuals, groups of persons, and great nations. China has appreciated this principle over most of its long history. Classical scholars knew the importance of stimulation and encouragement from others, and the Han, Tang, and Ming emperors, to varying degrees, fostered links with other peoples and cultures.

In the modern world, domestically derived ideas and perceptions alone are insufficient to ensure the safety and security of a way of life, much less of progress and modernization in any field, including medicine. Our country's fate under the Qing dynasty testified to this all too clearly. Even the relatively short moratorium on international contact during the 1960s and early 1970s cost our country very dearly. I hope that we Chinese will never again return to a state of intellectual isolation under the guise of self-reliance.

With our present shortage of teachers, the programs of scholarly exchange with the outside world can probably do more good than any other attempt to upgrade the efficiency of our health system. What forms these programs should take is a matter that must be constantly evaluated, in China as in any other country.

It may or may not be appropriate for public health graduate students from the Western democracies to restrict their interest to a relatively narrow range of advanced theoretical topics. It is clearly inappropriate, however, for those from developing countries to do so. Their graduate education should equip them for attacking the commonplace health problems of the Third World, whose remedies lie in such areas as improved sanitation, nutrition, maternal and child health care, and communicable disease control.

A number of cooperative agreements between Western and Chinese institutions were signed in the first flush of newly reestablished relations with the United States; however, there have been fewer as the fever subsided. In general, their full potential has not been realized because of difficulties at various levels of implementation. A fairly well established consensus in the mid-1980s seemed to hold that with limited resources on both sides, the focus should be on an exchange of individual scholars.

Two points in this context deserve some attention. First, when foreign scholars come to a developing country to study or teach in its health system, the value of their contribution in most instances has some proportion to the length of their stay. Even a brief visit may be quite beneficial to scholars for their own purposes. Yet, unless a scholar is prepared to remain for five years or longer, it is very difficult to surmount cultural barriers or to gain an in-depth perception of the problem under study; thus, the visiting scholar will be disappointed in not being able to contribute as fully as hoped. The foreign missionaries who came to China to study and teach before liberation in 1949 seemed to have appreciated the difficulty as many chose to spend their entire working lives in our country.

Second, when developing country medical students do graduate work abroad, the value of their experience to their country depends greatly on the topic on which they spend their research time. Too often such students are guided into areas of narrow research interest in highly technical areas. What the Third World needs is not so much people with greatly advanced specialized scientific medical knowledge, but medical and health professionals trained to respond to chronic, common problems, especially the common health problems in their own countries. Emphasis on advanced technology and specialized research in medical education and practice may serve the industrialized countries well—although even there it is evident that accelerating costs are an unwanted side effect. For students from developing countries, however, it is indisputably inappropriate.

ISSUES FOR THE FUTURE

Where do we go from here? The people of my country, of whom more than 80 percent are farmers, represent more than one-fifth of the total population of the world. That figure lends global significance to both our past experience in rural health development and the future direction of our health endeavors. What happens in China will have crucial implications on the level of "health for all in the year 2000."

In retrospect, we see that in China the expansion of the rural health infrastructure since 1958 has brought conspicuous, tangible benefits to our farmers. The increase in access to modern medical care in the countryside is, in fact, nothing short of remarkable. Every county in China, no matter how remote, now offers some form of scientific medical care to its inhabitants. County facilities not only exist but are being used extensively. Xiang centers, employing both modern and traditional methods, are treating a great volume of patients. The familiarity of attending physicians with the personal situations and problems of their neighbors and friends enhances the quality of the physician–patient relationship. Meanwhile, in the villages, barefoot doctors and village health workers, notwithstanding their need for further training and closer supervision, are rendering a very important service, essentially doing primary health care and preventive work.

Medical care, of course, is just one of the influences on health; the total health experience in China is a combination of external circumstances together with improved curative and preventive care that resulted in the striking health improvements since liberation in 1949. Educational and health improvements played a significant role; no one as yet has made a scientific examination of the probable correlation between higher family income and improved nutrition. Yet, it is fairly safe to assume that parents are spending some of their added income on better food for the children. Education has contributed to improved habits of cleanliness among the farmers, helping to reduce the prevalence of diarrhea and trachoma, often associated with poor personal hygiene. It has also made the peasants more conscious of the potential for infection and more interested in maintaining a sanitary environment.

The most critical determinant of development in health, as in all other realms of the national life, however, has been the centralization of political authority in the CCP and the government. The countrywide extension of the rural health infrastructure could never have been accomplished at so swift a pace and might never have been accomplished except in the distance future, had it not been for the strong backing of the Communist party and its then party chairman.

Absolute authority provided other advantages for improving the national health situation as well. For example, the government can encourage top students to attend medical school and can distribute them among the various medical training institutions in the manner most advantageous to the country. Also, after their graduation, it could send them to work where they were needed, rather than where they necessarily preferred to work, although there was some leverage for individual choice within the system.

Given what we have already been able to do, perhaps no other country has a better opportunity than China now enjoys to refine and elaborate a really outstanding health service from which other nations may draw inspiration. If quality and quantity are kept in balance, continuous penetration of scientific medical knowledge and skill into the everyday lives of our millions of villagers is all but guaranteed. It is a chance that we do not want to waste.

All in all, we have made a promising effort. Our level of health has been significantly improved, and we have an infrastructure in place, fully staffed. I believe that the next step is enlarging the promise by raising the quality of service. This raises several important issues, including the need for further training of local health personnel.

In any scheme to improve training, provincial authorities should, in my view, accept responsibility for improving the skills of county-level health personnel, who should be sent to provincial hospitals and clinics for this purpose. A selected few county health workers might even be enrolled in key medical schools or sent abroad for advanced study if that were deemed necessary.

My strong conviction, however, is that the most of the retraining of rural health workers should be done right in the rural areas, as the responsibility of county and xiang authorities. If country doctors, secondary medical school graduates, or rural nurses are sent to the city for training, they will be apt to seek means to avoid returning to the countryside. Conversely, the diversion of urban personnel to rural areas for service would serve no useful purpose either, since—unused to village conditions and uninterested in rural problems—they would soon become restless. In any event, there are plenty of candidates for remedial training already in the ranks of local rural health personnel.

Time and effort need not be spent on the construction of new educational facilities, as existing hospitals, maternal and child health centers, antiepidemic stations, and training schools can serve the purpose quite adequately. What is required of the existing training schools is that they maintain academically rigorous standards. Also, a program to bring more uniformity in the length and substance of training, at least in schools within each province, would go a long way toward ironing out some of the unevenness that now exists in the training of rural health personnel. Relatively uniform standards for the selection of students would also be helpful in this context.

Training schools should be given a modicum of suitable equipment, which need not be elaborate. This might include a tape recorder, a microscope, a centrifuge, a refrigerator, an incubator, and scales. A model training school in one selected county, appropriately equipped and staffed by dedicated teachers comfortable in a rural assignment, might draw favorable attention from other county authorities.

Implicit in these ideas is the underlying idea that secondary medical school graduates and country doctors should be given an opportunity to learn more about what they are already doing, and not that the scope of their responsibilities should be expanded. For example, the country doctors and village health workers are already doing effective immunization work. Yet it would be helpful to the program if those administering the vaccines understood more about why they produce immunity, what side effects may result, how long the immunity lasts, and why only a certain number of immunizations are given. Or, as another example, more emphasis should be given in the training programs to symptoms of communicable disease, especially infectious disease, which may be more widespread in rural areas than we realize.

The continuing education programs for local health personnel that are most urgently needed, then, are those that will further qualify physicians and village health workers to carry out preventive programs, to treat common ailments without producing harmful side affects, and to identify cases of communicable disease at an early stage so that the patients can be hospitalized immediately and the spread of infection to others prevented.

As long as workers in this category are performing relatively limited functions, simple first aid work, and vaccination, they are fulfilling an important service in many cases. When they are permitted to engage in curative practice, however, prescribing any drugs for any patient, the stage is set for problems.

For instance, with little or no training, a country doctor, failing to understand the source of the problem, may all too easily administer morphine to relieve the acute abdominal pain of a patient suffering from appendicitis, with the result that the patient eventually suffers a ruptured appendix. Rather than trying to organize graduate training for practitioners of that type, it seems more appropriate to limit the scope of their activities and leave the skilled work to others with appropriate training.

More difficult to solve are economic issues, the question of how country doctors might be appropriately remunerated, and how state medicine might eventually be brought to the xiang level and below. The solution of the former question in terms of letting country doctors engage in private practice is fraught with many difficulties, already cited. These questions need to be further studied.

Another matter of great consequence in our health future lies in the area of prevention. In my view, there is a very urgent need to tighten up supervision by the xiang-level authorities of the immunization work being done in the villages, so as to ensure quality control.

The village is the place where immunization work has been done and should be done. Nevertheless, village-level personnel seldom fully understand the scientific principles inherent in the immunization procedure. Therefore, they can make serious mistakes that undermine the value of the entire prevention campaign. They may, for example, fail to appreciate the importance of age as a criterion for immunization and immunize members of the wrong age group, or they may not understand the importance of proper vaccine storage. UNICEF has made a major contribution to child health in the Third World with its development and distribution of equipment to maintain vaccine at proper temperatures while it is in transit to the villages. So that full advantage is taken of that concept, however, xiang-level personnel who know so much more about the scientific fundamentals of a vaccination program absolutely must work in close cooperation with the village personnel. Unless the vaccination efforts are continuous, their long-term value will be lost.

Improved education of public health specialists is another issue that needs further study in our country. As noted earlier, public health education as modeled after the Soviet system currently emphasizes topical discussion, for example, of physical elements in the human environment, and performance of laboratory experiments rather than the application of scientific knowledge to common health problems. In my view, a shift away from the theoretical toward the more practical side of the public health field, particularly if field training were more widely used, would be of greater benefit to the country and would perhaps attract a higher quality student to the public health field.

In moving our health care approach farther along the road toward a population-based system that combines curative and preventive procedures, we would be making an important step in providing more fieldwork to public health students. Work could be coordinated systematically with the health service organizations at the county, xiang, and village levels. Some of our health centers (antiepidemic stations) offer facilities that would be excellent field training sites, especially for communicable disease control, health education, and school health.

Public health education in medical colleges in China could be strengthened as well; as long as good teachers are in short supply, the organization of separate schools of public health within the universities of medical sciences may be unwise. In particular, public health teaching to medical students could be made more effective by building a field training capability into our medical service. As long as the faculty themselves have no field experience, the teaching of public health or community medicine is bound to be largely classroom work sprinkled with some simple, even trivial, laboratory exercises. Yet as long ago as in my preliberation work at Xiaozhuang, my experience taught me that medical students in public health benefit less by didactic instruction than by participation in practical field activities.

Clinical instruction cannot be satisfactory without a good teaching hospital; public health teaching cannot be successful without a good teaching field. In the rural areas, students become inspired by direct contact with people; they begin to try to apply what they have learned to the solution of social problems; they see how problems can be handled through skillful organization and resourceful use of available technology; and they learn how to assess health conditions from the multiple perspectives of medicine, economics, education, sociology, and politics. In sum, in the field, they reorient their interests to the real needs of the people.

A good teaching hospital cannot be organized without compassionate effort by the staff, who consider medical problems for the benefit of all patients. Likewise, a good teaching field for public health education cannot be created except by a dedicated faculty with creative ideas and high ideals.

Underlying all this is the urgent need to instill a more community-oriented mentality in the next generation of physicians in our country. In my view, it is critically important that we make a greater effort to nurture young physicians who are public health-minded, that is, whose professional perspective is oriented on the community as a whole or that at least combines concern both for individuals and for the community.

For two reasons, this is essential not only for us, in China, but for countries throughout the world. First, universally, there are far greater numbers of medical students than of public health students. Consequently, once they enter the health field, their collective influence will be greater, and they can contribute just as much, or more, to the protection of the public at large as can the public health specialists. Second, it is medical school graduates, certainly in our country if not elsewhere, rather than public health school graduates, who come to occupy most of the administrative positions in the health system. Thus, if we are interested in the organization of a good health system, we must not fail to imbue our future administrators with an understanding and appreciation of community medicine. So far in China we have not done very much in that regard, and that is why the preventive aspect of our health picture has received less attention than some persons might have hoped.

Public health as a general field, particularly public health education, is a subject that has not elicited great interest in our country in recent years. In this respect, however, China is no different from many countries in the West. In many countries around the world, few people understand or are concerned about the meaning of the concept of public health. This is perfectly reasonable since many are struggling simply to secure the essentials of life.

In the industrialized West, however, where the term "public health" was coined, the level of affluence and education should be sufficient to ensure a different situation. One would hope to find not only that the abstract meaning of public health was generally understood but also that the significance of efforts to promote it were recognized and respected. Such is not necessarily the case, however. Even in medical circles in the West, one often encounters a somewhat disparaging attitude toward physicians in the public health field. It will be a change for the better when community medicine and public health are as respected as the branches of medicine on which individual clinical practice is based.

A CLOSING COMMENT

It may be that a scientifically based system of health care for an entire population can evolve only in stages as a public perception of social responsibility increases. In a progressive society, health care eventually becomes a function of collective concern about all circumstances and conditions that at all times affect the well-being of the entire group rather than of the concern of a single physician seeking a cure for an individual patient. Along with this, there is a shift away from reliance on curative measures alone and toward the use of both preventive and curative measures.

To my way of thinking, four stages can be identified in this process: individualized medicine, with attention only to curative measures; individualized medicine, with attention to both curative and preventive measures; community medicine; and, finally, public health.

Community medicine, the third and relatively advanced stage, and the one at which China is currently developing its health care approach, entails organized community efforts in medicine and health, using combined curative and preventive techniques. Because it is population-based, that is, based on the needs and conditions of communities as a whole, it encompasses almost by definition, the fields of vital statistics, epidemiology, and health administration.

Public health carries the scientific approach to health care to its ultimate point. As I define it, it is a field concerned with the entire range of circumstances and conditions that affect the health of an entire population. Preventive medicine is the stronger of its two components; in its curative component, the emphasis is on early diagnosis. Given the many circumstances that directly or indirectly impact the health and well-being of a population, public health is closely linked to many other scientific fields, particularly engineering and education.

These close linkages attest to the need to seek health care improvements in conjunction with other measures and programs to improve popular well-being. For this reason medicine and medical scientists, especially in developing countries, cannot afford to be absorbed in technology alone, least of all isolated in laboratory research efforts. The education of young physicians for our needs must be focused on, not detached from, reality.

In a medical school, all too often both teachers and students are interested in technology. In terms of its application and development for the benefit of the general population, however, not many are interested. Yet medicine, after all, deals with human beings. So, in a country where pioneer leadership in health is badly needed, an initial step may be to rely heavily on those medical students who are sensitive to social needs and who have had some training in the liberal arts and humanities, for it is they who are more likely to think in terms of social well-being in the broad sense.

Such persons can be relied on to find an appropriate means of bringing health care to less advantaged segments of Asian, African, and Latin American societies. Large-scale extension of health services, however, is perhaps best avoided until the model on which it is based has proved practical on a local scale. Local communities cannot be expected to progress in health care delivery, regardless of how good the model, without strong support from government or other outside agencies; they are simply too fragile. Firm central government effort is probably needed in every situation.

Whatever the specific nature of the delivery system that evolves, it should be marked by strong organization and integration at every level. It needs good administration at the top and enthusiastic workers, including lay workers, at the bottom. Clearly delineated technical and professional distinctions contribute to the coherence of the system. The contribution of education and training programs in this regard is self-evident. In every country continuing education to all technical personnel is crucial. The competency of the teachers is essential, for their role has much to do with determining the educational outcome.

Much can be gained through international exchange and foreign assistance, provided the focus of this assistance is appropriate. Acceptance of scientific equipment from abroad that local personnel know neither how to operate nor to maintain may not be very helpful. It is better that international assistance be directed toward better training of medical personnel and toward the expansion of the scientific horizons of the national leadership, possibly through foreign-sponsored visits to other countries or through international conferences.

Centuries have passed since people first began to organize themselves into nations. Each nation has had its own particular concerns,
but all have been concerned with medical and health care. Now, in
1988, concern with "Health for all by the year 2000" becomes an
appeal on behalf of all humankind. The response must come from
people in many fields of endeavor, across the entire spectrum of
society. Yet, in helping nature to protect and promote human
health, the medical profession must bear the primary responsibility.

All this may sound banal, but even ideas based in common
sense are often difficult to realize. I shall look back satisfied if I see
that the far-sighted teachings of the past continue to flourish in the
minds of younger colleagues and friends. Most of China's problems, medical and social, and probably those of the rest of the
world as well, can be understood from a historical point of view. I
hope that the contemporary history of my own country will be a
source of pride for future generations.

"Birth, aging, sickness, and death" constitutes a life cycle, a
biological law that no one can resist. Everyone desires to live long
and well. Nature aids us in this context, in both health and illness,
and medicine, a body of knowledge accumulated by humankind, is
there to assist. As the stewards of this knowledge, physicians have
a special responsibility to persons struggling to realize their human
rights in regard to health.

In many parts of the world, the vast majority of people are beset
by poverty, ignorance, and illness. The medical profession must
join the fight to combat these afflictions. When it does not, or
worse still, even aggravates these circumstances (when some physicians take advantage of their special knowledge at the expense of
such persons), something has gone wrong in that society. In a just
society, medical care of good quality should be easily available to
all the people.

Notes

1: ENCOUNTER BETWEEN TWO MEDICINES

1. Albert Feuerwerker, "Economic Trends in the Later Ch'ing Empire, 1870–1911," in *The Cambridge History of China*, Denis Twitchett and John K. Fairbank, genl. eds., vol. 11, part 2, *Late Ch'ing, 1800–1911*, Kwang-Ching Liu and John K. Fairbank, eds. (London: Cambridge University Press, 1980), 4.

2. Rinn-Sup Shinn, "Historical Setting," in *China: A Country Study*, Frederica M. Bunge and Rinn-Sup Shinn, eds. (Washington, D.C., Government Printing Office, 1981), 14–15.

3. Ibid., 3–4.

4. Pierre M. Perrolle, "Science and Technology," in *China: A Country Study*, 295.

5. Shinn, "Historical Setting," 19.

6. Ibid., 19.

7. Perrolle, "Science and Technology," 295.

8. Shinn, "Historical Setting," 21.

9. Ibid., 23.

10. The basis for this discussion of indigenous medicine comes from Wen-lan Fan, *A Concise History of China*, 2 vols., 1: 1954, 73, 78; 2: 1957, 9, 30.

11. Shinn, "Historical Setting," 9.

12. For an interesting discussion of objectives and methods of the medical missionaries, see Paul U. Unschuld, *Medicine in China: A History of Ideas* (Berkeley, Los Angeles, London: University of California Press, 1985), 235–243.

13. Ibid., 238.

14. Ibid., 239.

15. John K. Fairbank, Edwin O. Reischauer, and Albert M. Craig, *East Asia: Tradition and Transformation* (Boston: Houghton Mifflin, 1973), 307.

2: IDEAS AND IDEALS: MEDICAL
STUDENTS AND SOCIAL CHANGE

1. James E. Sheridan, "The Warlord Era: Politics and Militarism under the Peking Government, 1916–1928," in *The Cambridge History of China*, Denis Twitchett and John K. Fairbank, genl. eds., vol. 12, part 1, *Republican China, 1912–1949*, John K. Fairbank, ed. (London: Cambridge University Press, 1983), 284–322.

2. John B. Grant, "Rural Public Health" (mimeographed paper, n.p., n.d.).

3. Unschuld, *Medicine in China: A History of Ideas* (Berkeley, Los Angeles, London: University of California Press, 1985), 247.

4. Albert Feuerwerker, "The Foreign Presence in China," in *The Cambridge History of China*, vol. 12, part 1, *Republican China, 1912–1949* (London: Cambridge University Press, 1983), 176.

5. Unschuld, *Medicine in China: A History of Ideas*, 241.

6. C. C. Chen, "Call on a Sick Friend," *The Binying Weekly* (Peking, 1: 1926: 221–224.

7. The reader interested in historical development of science and technology policy will find an informative discussion in Pierre M. Perrolle, "Science and Technology," in *China: A Country Study*, 294–297.

8. Mary Brown Bullock, *An American Transplant: The Rockefeller Foundation and Peking Union Medical College.* (Berkeley, Los Angeles, London: The University of California Press, 1980), 20, 80.

9. John B. Grant, "Chain Reaction in the Social Development of Health Care Services: The Chinese Example" (mimeographed paper, n.p., n.d.), 2.

10. Shinn, Rinn-Sup, "Historical Setting," 24.

11. C. C. Chen, "Concurrent Problems of Medicine, Public Health and Pharmacy," *The Binying Weekly* (Peking, 1926), 1: 210–219; 2: 89–110.

12. Ibid. (1927), 1: 221–224.

13. Ibid. (1929), 4: 21–23.

14. Ibid. (1929), 4: 1–3, 34.

15. Ibid. (1928), 2: 291–294.

16. Ibid. (1928), 2: 75–81.

17. Ibid. (1928), 3: 44–47.

18. Ibid. (1928), 3: 47.

19. Ibid. (1927), 1: 54–57.

20. Ibid. (1929), 4: 21–23.

21. Ibid. (1928), 2: 291–294.

22. Ibid. (1928), 2: 75–81.

23. Ibid. (1929), 4: 21–23.

24. Ibid. (1928), 3: 44–47.

25. Ibid. (1927), 1: 54–57.

3: PIONEERING IN RURAL HEALTH
DEVELOPMENT

1. Rinn-Sup Shinn, "Historical Setting," in *China: A Country Study*, 24–26.
2. Jean Chesneaux, Francoise Le Barbier, and Marie-Claire Bergere, *China from the 1911 Revolution to Liberation* (New York: Pantheon Books, 1977), 155–183 passim.
3. C. C. Chen, *The Binying Weekly* (Peking, 1926), 4: 21–23.

4: MEDICINE AND HEALTH UNDER
WARTIME CONDITIONS

1. Mary Brown Bullock, *An American Transplant: The Rockefeller Foundation and Peking Union Medical College* (Berkeley, Los Angeles, London: The University of California Press, 1980), 159.

5: THE HEALTH EXPERIENCE IN THE 1949–
1976 PERIOD

1. A discussion of Soviet influence on scientific research and policy-making institutions appears in Pierre M. Perrolle, "Science and Technology," in *China: A Country Study*.

6: A NEW ERA IN HEALTH DEVELOPMENT

1. An informative discussion of the process entailed in the implementation of reform guidelines may be found in Robert L. Suettinger, "The Political Process," in *China: A Country Study*, 371–381.
2. These data are taken from a county health report issued by Shifang County authorities in 1986.
3. Ibid.
4. Ibid.
5. Ibid.

Selected Bibliography

Bowers, John Z. *Western Medicine in a Chinese Palace: Peking Union Medical College, 1917–1951.* Philadelphia: The Josiah Macy, Jr. Foundation, 1972.

Bullock, Mary Brown. *An American Transplant: The Rockefeller Foundation and Peking Union Medical College.* Berkeley, Los Angeles, London: University of California Press, 1980.

Ch'en, C. C. "Civilization, Knowledge, and Medicine." *The Binying Weekly* (Peking) 1 (1926): 2–4.

———— "Water Supply of Peking." *The Binying Weekly* (Peking) 1 (1926): 208–209.

———— "Concurrent Problems of Medicine, Public Health and Pharmacy." *The Binying Weekly* (Peking) 1 (1926): 210–219.

———— "Discussion of Various Problems in Medicine." *The Binying Weekly* (Peking) 1 (1926): 219–222.

———— "Review of One Year of Publication. *The Binying Weekly* (Peking) 1 (1927): 54–57.

———— "Call on a Sick Friend." *The Binying Weekly* (Peking) 1 (1926): 221–224.

———— "Medical Reconstruction Problems of Our Country." *The Binying Weekly* (Peking). 2 (1928): 47.

———— "Objectives of Education." *The Binying Weekly* (Peking) 2 (1928): 65–67.

———— "The Economics of Health." *The Binying Weekly* (Peking) 2 (1928): 75–81.

———— "The Importance of Public Health Administration in Relation to General Education." *The Binying Weekly* (Peking) 2 (1928): 291–294.

———— "The Binying Medical Society and Its Functions." *The Binying Weekly* (Peking) 3 (1928): 1–5.

———— "Medical Organization for Protection of Our Community." *The Binying Weekly* (Peking) 3 (1928): 44–47.

———— "Hsiaochuang Rural Health Demonstration." *The Binying Weekly* (Peking) 3 (1929): 48–51.

———— "Rural Health and China's Education." *The Binying Weekly* (Peking) 4 (1929): 21–23.

———— "We Need State Medicine." *The Binying Weekly* (Peking) 4 (1929): 35.

———— "We Shall Soon Practice State Medicine." *The Binying Weekly* (Peking) 6 (1929): 34.

———— "The Tinghsien (Dingxian) Experiment in Medical Relief and Health Protection. Chinese Mass Education Movement (n.p.), 1933.

———— "A Practical Survey of Rural Health." *Chinese Medical Journal* (n.v.) (1933): 680–688.

———— "Sickness: An Important Cause of Absenteeism in Rural Schools." *Chinese Medical Journal* (n.v.) (1933): 594–596.

———— "Scientific Medicine as Applied in Tinghsien." *Milbank Memorial Fund Quarterly* 11 (1933): 370–378.

———— "Public Health in Rural Reconstruction at Tinghsien." *Milbank Memorial Fund Quarterly* 12 (1934): 370–378.

———— "An Experiment in Health Education in Chinese Country Schools." *Milbank Memorial Fund Quarterly* 12 (1934): 232–247.

———— "State Medicine and Medical Education. *Chinese Medical Journal* 49 (1935): 951–954.

———— "The Rural Public Health Experiment in Tinghsien." *Milbank Memorial Quarterly* 14 (1936): 66–80.

———— "The Development of Systematic Training in Rural Public Health Work in China." *Milbank Memorial Fund Quarterly* 14 (1936): 370–387.

———— "Some Problems of Medical Organization in Rural China." *Chinese Medical Journal* 51 (1937): 803–814.

Chesneaux, Jean, Francoise Le Barbier, and Marie-Claire Bergere. *China from the 1911 Revolution to Liberation.* New York: Pantheon Books, 1977.

Chia, Kwei. "What is Public Health?" *The Binying Weekly* (Peking) 1 (1926): 47.

Europa Publications Ltd. "China." In *The Far East and Australia*, 17th ed. London: Europea Publications, Ltd., 1985.

Fairbank, John K. Edwin O. Reischauer, and Albert M. Craig. *East Asia: Tradition and Transformation.* Boston: Houghton Mifflin, 1973.

Feuerwerker, Albert. "Economic Trends in the Later Ch'ing Empire, 1870–1911." In *The Cambridge History of China*, Denis Twitchett and John K. Fairbank, genl. eds., vol. 11, part 2, *Late Ch'ing, 1800–1911*, Kwang-Ching Liu and John K. Fairbank, eds. London: Cambridge University Press, 1980.

———— "The Foreign Presence in China." In *The Cambridge History of China*, vol. 12, part 1, *Republican China, 1912–1949*. London: Cambridge University Press, 1983.

Fraser, Robert, ed. *Keesings.* Item 33719B, vol. 31, no. 1. London: Longman Group Ltd., 1985.

Grant, James D. "An Analysis of the Objectives, Techniques, and Accomplishments of Dr. John B. Grant in Establishing the First Health Station of Peking, China." (Unpublished paper, 1973).

Grant, John B. "Rural Public Health." (Mimeographed paper, n.p., n.d.)

———— "The Horizontal Group Approach to Community Development." (Mimeographed paper, n.p., 1931.)

———— In *Health Care for the Community, Selected Papers,* Conrad Seipp, ed. Baltimore: Johns Hopkins University Press, 1963, pp. 148–153.

Hou, Hsiang-ch'uan, and Chih-Chi'ien Chen. "The Proteolytic Enzyme of Hsian-kua, Cucumis Melo, Linn." *Chinese Journal of Physiology* 1 (2) (1927): 33–36.

Kallgren, Joyce K. "China 1979: On Turning Thirty," *Asian Survey* 20 (1) (January 1980): 1–18.

———— "Sino-American Cultural Relations: Exchanges Reconsidered." (Unpublished paper presented at the Regional Seminar in Chinese Studies, Center for Chinese Studies, University of California, Berkeley, April 12–13, 1985.)

Li, Ching-han. Chapter 6 "Health and Sanitation." In *General Survey of Tinghsien.* (n.p.), 1933, chap. 6, pp. 219–283.

Lisowski, Pere. "The Emergence and Development of the Barefoot Doctor in China." *The Journal of the Japanese Society of Medical History* 25 (1979): 339–392.

Lucas, AnElissa. "Changing Medical Models in China: Organizational Options or Obstacles?" *China Quarterly* 83 (September 1980): 480–489.

New, Peter Kong-ming, and New, Mary Louise. "The Barefoot Doctors of China: Healers for All Seasons." In *Culture, Disease and Healing,* David Landy, ed. New York: Macmillan, 1974.

———— and Cheung, Yuet-wah. "An Examination into the Roots of Health Care Delivery in the People's Republic of China." Paper presented at the Politics of Health Conference, Bethune College, York University, Downsview, Ontario, April 15, 1979. (Mimeographed.)

———— "Third World Medicine and Social Change." In *The People's Republic of China: A Socio-Historical Examination of its \Health Care Delivery,* John H. Morgan, ed. University Press of America (no location given), 1983, pp. 173–186.

———— "Integrating Traditional and Western Medicine in the People's Republic of China: Policy Issues in Its Socio-Historical Context." Paper presented at a meeting of the Southern Anthropological Society (no location given), April 19, 1984.

Oksenberg, Michael, ed. *China's Developmental Experience,* New York: Praeger, 1973.

Perrolle, Pierre M. "Science and Technology." In *China: A Country Study,* Frederica M. Bunge and Rinn-Sup Shinn, eds. Washington, D.C.: Government Printing Office, 1981, pp. 291–322.

Sheridan, James E. "The Warlord Era: Politics and Militarism under the Peking Government, 1916–1928." In *The Cambridge History of China*, Denis Twitchett and John K. Fairbank, genl. eds. vol. 12, part 1, *Republican China, 1912–1949*, John K. Fairbank, ed. London: Cambridge University Press, 1983, pp. 284–322.

Shinn, Rinn-Sup. "Historical Setting." In *China: A Country Study*, Frederica M. Bunge and Rinn-Sup Shinn, eds. Washington, D.C.: Government Printing Office, 1981, pp. 1–42.

Sichuan Medical College, School of Public Health Administration, Department of Community Medicine, and Sichuan School of Continuing Education. "A Study of Primary Health Care in Shifang County, Sichuan Province." 1983. (Author anonymous.)

———— "An Analysis of Health Personnel Status in Sichuan Province." 1984. (Author anonymous.)

Sidel, Ruth, and Victor W. Sidel. "The Political Pendulum, 1971–1981" and "Shoes for the Barefoot Doctor?" In *The Health of China*. Boston: Beacon Press, 1982, pp. 3–16, 35–70.

Suettinger, Robert L. "The Political Process." In *China: A Country Study*, Frederica M. Bunge and Rinn-Sup Shinn, eds. Washington, D.C.: Government Printing Office, 1981, pp. 353–394.

Unschuld, Paul U. *Medicine in China: A History of Ideas*. Berkeley, Los Angeles, London: University of California Press, 1985.

Wang, Teh-chen. *An Analysis of Utilization of Medical and Health Services in Tunghsien*. Peking: The School of Traditional Medicine, 1984.

White, Kerr Lachian. "Life, Death and Medicine: With Bibliographic Sketch." *Scientific American* 229 (9) (1973): 22–23.

World Health Organization. "Global Strategy for Health for all by the Year 2000." *Health for All, Series 3*. Geneva: World Health Organization, 1981.

Yang, C. S. "Editorial." *The Binying Weekly* (Peking) 1 (1926): 1.

Yen, Y. C. James. *The Tinghsien Experiment in 1934*. Silang, Cavite, the Philippines: The International Institute of Rural Reconstruction, 1975, 40 pp.

Yip, Ka-che. "Health and Society in China: Public Health Education for the Community, 1912–1937 [American Medical Missionaries]." *Social Science and Medicine* 16 (12) (1982): 1197–2005.

———— "Medicine and Nationalism in the People's Republic of China." *Canadian Review of Studies in Nationalism* (n.v.) (1983): 175–185.

In addition to the above sources, a number of other works in Chinese and English were consulted. These included a number of surveys, conference reports, and periodical articles, both published and unpublished, omitted because complete citations could not be provided or because the works are unlikely to be available in libraries outside China. Some material in this volume also is drawn from personal conversations and private correspondence.

Designer: U.C. Press Staff
Compositor: Huron Valley Graphics
Text: 10/13 Palatino
Display: Palatino
Printer: Braun-Brumfield, Inc.
Binder: Braun-Brumfield, Inc.